MW01537924

Witness to the Dark

My Daughter's Troubled Times
A Comedy of Emotions

Bob Larsted

Witness to the Dark:
My Daughter's Troubled Times. A Comedy of Emotions.
by Bob Larsted

Copyright © 2013 Bob Larsted
All rights reserved

Contact the author at bob@boblarsted.com
Visit my website at www.boblarsted.com

Portions Copyright © Patricia Larsted. Used with permission.
Who Am I in 5 Steps form Copyright © Quinsigamond Community
College, Worcester, Massachusetts. Used with permission.
Cover photograph by Laurence Delderfield.
Author caricature by Keelan Parham, www.KeelanParham.com.

Some of the names and identifying characteristics of persons and places
discussed in this book have been changed to protect their identities.
At the request of his father, Gregg, Brian Sculthorpe's name is unchanged.

A Note to the Reader:
The information contained in this book is not intended to serve as a
replacement for professional medical advice. Any use of the information
in this book is at the reader's discretion. The author and publisher
specifically disclaim any and all liability arising directly or indirectly from
the use or application of any information contained in this book. A health
care professional should be consulted regarding your specific situation.

Published in Holden, Massachusetts, United States of America

Library of Congress Control Number: 2012908192

ISBN: 9781468150131

2 4 6 8 9 7 5 3 1

Table of Contents

A Note from My Daughter, Patricia, at Age 20

My father used to be shy. He came to all my medical appointments, but never talked to the doctors. He drove me to my friends' houses, but never spoke with their parents. He went to PTA meetings, but never opened his mouth. Maybe, if nothing else, the good that came out of my illness and recovery is that he has found his voice. He has written this book, effectively speaking to anyone courageous enough to read it.

My father is analytical. I'm the artsy one. I write poetry. It's something I've been doing ever since eighth grade when a supportive teacher helped me find my voice. Through poetry, I can vent to a piece of paper without worrying about what it thinks of me, or if it will tell anyone about the darkness I was stuck in for years before I finally found some light. Today's poems are brighter.

I'd always thought I would be the one in my family to write a book. It never occurred to me my father would write one, especially before I mine. He told me about his book when I was nineteen and doing better, when he asked my permission to tell his view of my story. He asked to use some of my poetry. I was flattered. Find his favorites sprinkled throughout this book. Find my favorites in my book, *Of Meadows and Flowers: and Crying and Hope*.

People ask me how I feel about him writing about me, telling the world my deep, dark secrets. Things I was reluctant to tell him. Things that only came out after years of therapy. I was never nervous. His writing has opened my eyes to my own messed-up world, and how it, and I, affect those around me.

Reading this, I have seen my life through the eyes of another. And that's an amazing thing to be able to do, something only famous people usually get to do. Does that make me famous? I don't particularly want to be, and please don't stop me on the street, but maybe, someday, my story will save a shy or lonely teen's life. And every life is worth saving.

My father sees things differently than others. This book was not written to be artsy, it was written to prove a point — that we were able to get through this, and everyone else deserves that same chance.

At the back of this book, in the Lessons Learned chapter, there is advice for parents, teachers, and some others who should pay attention. I like the part for survivors. But it is missing one whole section. One giving advice to friends. When I told him this, he said he wasn't qualified. And that I should write it. Here is what it should say:

Look out for your friends. Because if mine had realized how messed up I was in sixth grade when I was saying that I wanted to find a way to fall off the edge of the world, it would have saved me two years of being depressed and alone.

Be tough, and remember, recovery is real.

—Patricia Larsted, January 2013

Preface

I'm Bob. My wife Kate and I are proud parents of two perfect children. Beth, the younger, is doing a remarkable job of thriving and surviving her adolescence among the chaos that defines our family. Patricia, her no-longer-quite-so-suicidal sister, has managed to make it through her teens. For quite some time, it seemed as if she might not. This book is my take on our journey together through those frightening years.

The first hint I ever had that I wanted to be a writer was the day I finished my first letter to the Environmental Protection Agency. I had to explain to them why we had just failed a particularly important air-emissions test on a new piece of equipment at my workplace. By the time my letter was done, I had convinced myself that because of that unsuccessful test, the world was going to be a better and cleaner place than if we had passed.

I appreciate technology and all it can do for us. I enjoy the search for a well-engineered solution for whatever needs doing. Like our children, that emission-control system was supposed to work just fine when it came from the factory. But life doesn't always work out that way. I spent weeks redesigning and rebuilding the whole thing. I kept meticulous notes and documented all my changes. Incredibly, when the EPA inspector came back for the retest, he agreed that what we had come up with was far better and more reliable than what we started with.

For me, writing this book has been a Quest. It began at a time when things weren't going particularly well with Patricia. It wasn't clear what we should do. Patricia has been through much. This has taken significantly longer than weeks, and we still aren't done, but both she and I have changed dramatically because of what we have been through.

I always hoped that writing this book would give me the clarity to understand our journey. Maybe I could sum it all up in a quick letter to the world; the answers to her problems. I would finally understand what was important and what was just a part of her being. But once again, it hasn't worked out that way. What I've ended up with is this long and convoluted story. The answers remain clouded. But that's what it is like living with someone struggling to come to terms with her own mental health.

If you are a parent sharing a similar journey, or a friend or professional trying to be supportive, you know it's tough. It's relentless. Let's begin.

—Bob Larsted, January 2013

To Patricia
You make me so proud.

Witness to the Dark

My Daughter's Troubled Times
A Comedy of Emotions

Please, Dad. Help me.
Dry my tears.
Please, Dad. Help me.
Sedate my fears.

Please, Dad. Help me.
I can't stop crying.
Please, Dad. Help me.
I'm afraid of dying.

Dad, dear. Save me.
I feel so lost.
Dad, please. Save me.
Whatever the cost.

I'm sad and crying.
I just can't stop.
I'm really not lying.
This poem's a flop.

—Patricia

Confessions

If I weren't so tired, it would have been a good day to think about how much better things were going. It was Tuesday night. The dishes were done. The house was getting cleaner. Kate was in the other room watching reruns. Yesterday was Memorial Day. Summer was getting near. I sat in my chair—my recliner—something I hadn't been able to do for months. My older daughter, 14-year-old Patricia, came by and sat on the floor next to me. She put her head on my arm. My eyes closed. Life was good.

Then, she told me.

"Dad, I took some pills."

She told me she took some pills. *What?* "Pain pills. From the medicine cabinet." *When?* "A few months ago. December. After mom's stroke." *Why?* "I don't know. But I'm feeling better now." *How many pills?* "Fourteen." *What happened?* "I woke up the next morning with a headache." *Why?* "I don't know.

"And I cut myself.

"On my ankles. But I stopped. I'm feeling better now. That's why I told you. I'm OK now. I just wanted you to know."

Thank you for telling me.

∞

I remember the day many years earlier. I was a bachelor living in my new home—a fixer-upper—caught in the spiral of an ever-snowballing home-renovation nightmare going nowhere. I came in from work to find the house cold. Again. Automatically, I went down cellar to the oil burner and pressed the reset button. The ignition spark had been failing recently. I'd even called the repairman a couple of times, but something was still wrong. So I pressed the reset button, as I had done so many times before.

Twenty minutes later, the radiators were still cold. That was unusual. I went back down and reset it again. But as my finger came off the button, I sensed that something was wrong. Something was different. A sound. The oil burner was already on. Instantly, I realized that this time, in addition to ignition spark, the safety shut-off had just joined the long list of things to fix. And while I had been upstairs freezing, fuel oil had been pumping into the combustion chamber of that rickety old boiler. Lots of it.

But this time, the spark didn't fail. It lit. Through the peephole, I could see the swollen, orange flames. And hitting the emergency-stop switch didn't suddenly un-light all that oil.

It continued to burn. But it didn't explode. Yet.

∞

I'd never called 911 in my life. Never intended to. It would be an imposition. Our town had a volunteer fire department. They're at home with their families. If they came, they'd be mad at me for pressing the button. "Why didn't you get it fixed?" *I tried.* "Why didn't you try again?" *I did.* "Why did you press the button?" *I don't know. It seemed like the right thing to do.*

If they came, they'd track their boots and hoses through the sawdust and sheetrock of this month's project. They'd take their axes to my asbestos-covered boiler, oil would leak into the floor, and I'd be left with a toxic-waste dump instead of my dream home.

I can handle this myself.

I grabbed my fire extinguisher, ran outside into the night, and looked up at the chimney. Plumes of black smoke. Lots of it. But it was dark outside. As long as none of my neighbors looked up, I'd never be discovered. Technically, those weren't flames coming out of the chimney, either. It was just the glow from the inferno three stories down. Back to the cellar. More orange flames. I watched it burn.

After a while we had a new sound: steam. Venting out of the radiators. They were starting to get hot. The pressure was building. It didn't take me long to figure out that the high-pressure cutoff-switch wasn't going to help. The burner wasn't on. Once the pressure builds enough, the safety valve will blow—unless it fails, too. Hot steam will flood the basement. Roasting me. My fire extinguisher. When the steam runs out, the boiler will melt down. Everything nearby will burst into flames. Maybe then they won't feel so put out if I call 911.

Ultimately, I did handle it myself. There really wasn't any question. I waited as long as I could, but when the pressure got too much, I just opened the firebox door, emptied my extinguisher in there, and slammed the door shut again. The fire went out.

But everything was still hot. There was a hissing sound as the leftover oil in the bottom of the furnace evaporated. And started up the chimney. And ignited again on the red-hot walls. That's when it exploded. There was a bang. The boiler door flew open. A rush of flames. Then, nothing. Steam sounds stopped. The clicking of the hot metal slowed. Silence. *Mission accomplished.*

I'd proven once again I could manage things myself.

But the house started to cool off. And by three a.m., I realized I really did need help. So I called the oil company. I got their answering machine: "If this is a real emergency, press 1 to page the on-call technician. To leave a message for our next business day, begin speaking after the beep." This wasn't an emergency. And I don't talk to answering machines. So I hung up.

Ultimately, I called back. And I left a message. But not before I practiced it a couple of times first. I explained that my oil burner— the one they had tried to fix a couple of times—had failed. It dumped oil all over itself and almost burned my house down. I don't trust it anymore, and I want another one. Please.

No one called me back.

I knew what time they opened in the morning. I gave them plenty of time. When I couldn't stand it any longer, I called again. The service manager answered. I told him my oil burner had tried to kill me, and I wanted a new one. He sent a technician. It was one of the guys who had tried to fix it before. I showed him the problem. He said that this happens all the time. That he knew just what to do. "Nothing to worry about." I asked if he had a new burner with him. "Oh, no. I'll just change a few parts and you'll be fine." *But I'm scared of the old one.*

I probably imagined this, but I'm sure he patted me on the back of the hand, told me that he was the professional, and said everything was going to be OK. After he left, I changed the batteries in the smoke detectors and slept with one eye open for five years.

∞

It was nearly 20 years later when I finally called 911.

It was easy.

It was 7:16 on a snowy Friday morning, December 16th. Kate, my wife, was up for the kids. I put them to bed. While she got them off to school, I got to snooze. It was a good deal.

Through my sleep, I heard a strange noise coming from the laundry room down the hall. Kate sometimes went in there in the morning to get something to wear from the dryer. But today, something was different. A sound. I investigated.

I found Kate slumped on the floor. One leg into some pants. She was making an unusual noise. It was talking, but it wasn't English. Her head was drooped. She was like a puddle, only taller. As I lifted up her head, it tipped over the other way. I couldn't keep it straight. I tried to lean her against the washing machine. But she drooped. I stood up, walked to the bedroom, and called 911. It was easy.

Something's wrong with my wife. I need an ambulance. "What's wrong?" *I don't know.*

I ran back to her. Still slumped. I tried to plump her up. Didn't work. I ran downstairs, opened the front door, and started moving furniture out of the way to clear a path to the second floor. Back upstairs. Kate was the same. The kids were still in their rooms, just getting up to get ready for school. I heard a door begin to open. I shouted at them to stay in their rooms. "Why?" *Something's wrong with mom.* "What?" *I don't know. Stay in your room.*

Within what seemed like only two minutes, Officer Gregg Sculthorpe arrived. He's the only local cop I know by name. We've known each other for years. He's been at the neighborhood cookouts. We'd cruised to Bermuda with his wife, son, and a bunch of friends just a couple of years earlier. He was the school resource officer at my kids' elementary school.

He came upstairs and spoke with Kate. "Hi Kate." *Hi,* but garbled. He looked at me and said, "Stroke." After my involuntary exhale, he went on, "Probably just a TIA, a 'mini-stroke.' They happen all the time. She'll be fine." The ambulance arrived a few minutes later; they packed her off to the hospital; and saved her life. It wasn't a TIA. It was a stroke. A bad one.

Calling 911 was easy.

∞

So what are you supposed to do when your kid tells you she tried to kill herself? But she's fine now? Call 911? No, probably not. Some professional? Sure.

These things must happen all the time. She'll be fine.

I thanked Patricia for telling me. I told her I loved her and I was glad she was all right. She went to bed.

I told Kate. She listened, and went back to her recovery.

I began my new life.

Ultimately, this book is going to be about suicide. It might be about other things, too, but it is going to be about the possibility of suicide. It has to be. But we're not ready to go there yet. At least not as it relates to my child. For now, we'll just leave it that she "took some pills." It sounds better. Less final. Less terrifying. More medical.

The next morning, I called her in sick from school. I wondered for a moment if I should call the principal and tell him what was going on. He had been wonderful after Kate's stroke: "Anything you need. We'll watch out for her." *No.* It was too soon.

I called the doctor's office. I said that Patricia needed to see Dr. Fitzgerald. Today. Dr. Fitzgerald. Her pediatrician. Not someone else. Patricia had told me she had taken some pills, and we needed to talk with the doctor about this. This morning would be fine.

I'd been to the pediatrician before. Apparently, I'm one of those unusual fathers who get dragged to the children's annual physicals by the strong-willed wife. It came in handy after Kate's stroke because everyone in the office already recognized me. We checked in at the window, paid our co-pay, and sat down to wait. It didn't take long. One of the nurses came out and ushered us into the back. We sat, and she asked why we were here. Patricia just sat there, eyes down. I tried to encourage her to talk. The nurse asked again. Patricia didn't say anything. I said Patricia admitted to me that she took some pills. The nurse asked if this were true. Patricia remained quiet. The nurse told Patricia she needed to speak up if they were going to help her. After a while, the doctor came in.

Dr. Fitzgerald asked what was going on. She said she noticed that the staff had cleared her schedule and given her some time with Patricia this morning. I said Patricia had admitted to me that she had taken some pills. *Oh. When did you take the pills?* "Last December." *How many?* "Fourteen." *Why?* "I don't know." During our time there, we determined that Patricia had taken 14 pain pills, Tylenol or Motrin, from the medicine cabinet at home. She had done this at bedtime, on Monday, December 19, three days after Kate's stroke. She was feeling overwhelmed. Everyone at school had been asking her about mom. "How is she doing?" "Is everything OK?" "Can I do anything for you?" Kids and teachers who had never talked to her were trying to smother her with kindness.

I sat there remembering my phone calls to the school that Monday: "We'll watch out for her. She'll be fine." She didn't expect to wake up that Tuesday. But she did. By then, the kids were up to speed on how mom was doing, we'd made it through a day of school, and it had just become clear to us that we were being adopted by our town. There were two lists of people who would cook for us: the PTA contingent and the Girl Scout crowd. There might be some infighting and we might be getting two dinners some days. Rides would be available to sporting events and scout meetings. Play dates could be arranged on a moment's notice so I could go spend time with Kate at the hospital. These were not things that were within my comfort zone to accept, but a droopy puddle can change you pretty quickly.

Back at the doctor's office, Dr. Fitzgerald took charge. She asked questions. Patricia sat there and sobbed quietly but answered them as best she could. Yes, she was safe. Yes, she was feeling better. Yes, she probably had been feeling a little sad. Dr.

Fitzgerald told us that lots of children go through this. The word "depression" came up. She asked how Kate was doing. Patricia's face brightened. As they were finishing up, Dr. Fitzgerald and Patricia made something called a "Contract for Safety," a verbal pact whereby they agreed that if Patricia was feeling unsafe, she would tell mom or dad. It's amazing how something so useless made me feel so comforted.

Dr. Fitzgerald wrote out a list of people to call. Therapists. We needed to see a therapist. *What's a therapist?* "Someone to talk to." She warned us that the end of the school year was a particularly popular time for therapists. We might have trouble getting an appointment. I like Dr. Fitzgerald's understated manner.

I dropped Patricia off at school on my way home.

∞

So, how do you choose a therapist? Back then I was a little naïve. I thought you went through some kind of selection process. Start by figuring out where they practice. Is it easy to get to? What about parking? Is it a safe neighborhood? Do they have interesting reading material in the waiting room? Stuff like that.

But we are looking for a therapist here. What is a therapist, anyway? Maybe it matters if they are any good. How could I figure that out? Ask someone? I'm not ready for that. Beyond the fact that I wouldn't know whom to ask, or what, I'm not willing to tell anyone, even someone I don't know, that I'm looking for a therapist for my child. "Why are you looking for a therapist?" *Because she took some pills.* Not there yet. So qualifications are off the list.

It took me a while to figure it out, but there were really only two criteria for selecting Patricia's first therapist:

1) Do they call you back?
2) Do they take your insurance?

Nothing else matters.

I chose the first woman on the list and called. No one answered. I got a machine: "You have reached the confidential voice mailbox of Blah Blah. If this is a real emergency, hang up and dial 911 or go to your nearest hospital emergency room. If this is a patient emergency and you need to speak with the on-call staff, hang up and dial pager number: 555-0132. Punch in your phone number at the beep. Someone will give you a call. But make sure you remove the block from your phone, or we won't be able to return your call. To leave a detailed message, begin speaking after the beep." This sounded vaguely familiar, only more ominous.

I hung up.

Remember the part about not being willing to tell anyone I'm looking for a therapist for my daughter? Well, apparently, this applies to answering machines as well.

I practiced. And practiced. Finally, I came up with a message I was willing to say out loud and called back. The second time through, the therapist's message is pretty long. There is plenty of time to chicken out. I did, at least once. Or twice. Or maybe more.

No one called me back.

I was getting really nervous. I was going to have to talk with someone. A person. Tell them I was looking for a therapist for my child. Because she had taken some pills. "Why?" *I don't know.*

Late morning turned to afternoon.

The children would be home from school in a couple of hours. How could I talk on the phone if the kids were in the house? Besides, I needed to use the bathroom. What if they called? Still no call. Patricia came home. Her sister came home. I was freaking out. Now I was hoping they wouldn't call.

My wish was granted. For a week. No one called back.

A week can be a long time. When the kids were in school, I hoped for a call. Not that I wanted to talk with someone, but I promised Dr. Fitzgerald I would. When the kids were home, I panicked every time the phone rang. Patricia's friend. Her sister's friend. My mother. What am I going to tell her? *Lots of children go through this. She'll be fine.* Not likely. (The telling my mother part.)

After a week, I called the therapist back and left another message. It wasn't any better than the first. I'd been too busy waiting for a call to be practicing my message-leaving skills. I left my cell phone number instead of the home number. That way, I could go to the bathroom. Or to work. Or to market. I was free.

The problem was she actually called me back. Now I had to talk. Again, not something I had spent any time thinking about.

We had a nice chat. We danced around the issue. "My daughter needs a therapist. She's been depressed." The therapist sounded concerned and genuinely interested. Finally, I needed to say it. I used the words "suicide attempt" and "pills." Not something a father wants to utter in the same sentence with "my daughter."

Maybe it was me, but it seemed as though the tone of the conversation changed. We were now talking about something real. Something important. Something scary. Maybe I could really get her some help. Maybe Patricia really would be fine.

The therapist told me she wasn't available.

When you call the oil burner guy, "I'm not available," isn't on the list of possible responses. Even though Dr. Fitzgerald warned me about having trouble finding someone, "I'm not available," wasn't on my list of possible responses now, either.

I got out Dr. Fitzgerald's list of candidates, checked my selection matrix for the second best positioned/reading-materialed therapist, called, and left another message.

During this time, Patricia and I hadn't spent a lot of time talking about her confessions. Now and then, I asked her how she was feeling. She said OK. School was finishing up. Patricia was on the verge of graduating from middle school. Her sister would be done with elementary school. There were concerts to put on. Dances to attend. Dresses to shop for. The stress level was going up. Scheduling an appointment with a therapist wasn't going to fit into our busy schedule.

And there was the problem of the science trip to Florida a few days after school got out. Every year, one of the middle school science teachers takes a bunch of eighth graders to Florida for five days of science fun. They ride Space Mountain with the lights on to learn about physics. They have lunch with an astronaut. Kayak in the Everglades. Dissect a dead shark. And swim with the dolphins. Patricia had been looking forward to this. She was going with her friends. What happens when the therapist's office calls back and makes an appointment for when she is in Florida? Will I be a bad parent if I refuse? Would I be a good parent if I cancelled the trip so she could make an appointment? *Probably not.*

Thankfully, none of this was a problem. Because the new pattern is that nobody calls you back. A week went by. And I made the difficult and frightening decision to wait until Patricia came home from Florida before calling the therapist again. Relief. And as long as we didn't make contact, Patricia still wasn't "sick." But during these few weeks, I was still tormented by the irrational thought that someone still might actually call me back.

It wasn't a problem. Patricia went to Florida.

She swam with dolphins.

Summer. Time to call again. Yup. Maybe tomorrow. Things were going so well. Patricia seemed to be in great spirits. The stress and the rush of school ending had faded. Life was good, again. Until.

Until one night, Patricia asked me, "Do you think I'm bipolar?"

Apparently, Patricia had been spending time doing research while I was enjoying the calm. *Uh. I don't know. What makes you ask?* Maybe it was time for me to be doing some research.

I left another message with the therapist's office. Incredibly, Mark Wilkins called back. He does intake. That means we meet with him, talk about what's going on, and he matches us with one of the therapists in his office. We danced around the issue for a while. I said "suicide attempt." He said fine. The rub was that in order to get an appointment within a reasonable time, we'd need to be willing to drive the extra miles to Gardner because nothing was available at the Worcester office closer to our home. Remember, he was second on the selection-criteria list because of location. *Fine.* Apparently, two weeks is a reasonable time. For a kid who took some pills. Whose father let her go off to Florida by herself. We made the appointment.

Now that we had a date, what was going to happen next? I had no idea. It would be nearly seven months after her suicide attempt. And two months since I first learned of it. Maybe she's better. What are we going to talk about? What does a therapist do? I thought back to our meeting with Dr. Fitzgerald: Patricia sat and sobbed. Maybe I'd better be prepared to say something. But what?

So I started on a Quest. A Quest to discover the one childhood event that drove Patricia to do this. If I could only find it, she'd be fine. I really hoped it didn't have anything to do with bad parenting. Or bad fathering.

I was doomed.

The Quest

I learned in engineering school that in order to accomplish something, first you identify the problem. Then you assemble all the pertinent facts. Next, you employ the scientific method to identify your solution. Test it. And you're done. Or something like that. It had been a while since college.

This particular solution has some problems of its own: I don't know what the problem is. I don't know what the facts are. And even if I knew the facts, I don't know which of them are important. The smart thing to do at this time might have been to give up and let the professionals deal with it. It worked with the oil burner, didn't it? But I'm not that smart. Instead, I decided to make a list of everything I knew, prioritize it, and hopefully, in the process, identify the one thing we'd done to screw up our kid. Maybe we'd have it all figured out before her appointment. Then we could cancel it.

∞

We'd always liked Patricia. She was a great kid. More than any parent could hope for. She was smart. Contemplative. She had interesting things to say. She read constantly. I take credit for this, because I'd read hundreds of books out loud to her and her sister. Real books. Big books. Interesting books. Books with real stories with real problems. *Uh-oh.* Maybe we'll come back to this.

It wasn't until Patricia's younger sister Beth grew up a little more that we realized just how perfect Patricia was. Patricia never talked back. Never argued. She was helpful. If you asked a question, you got an answer. We learned later, just about three years later—because that's how much younger Beth is—that these are not typical qualities of an adolescent. Apparently, adolescents are loud and obnoxious. Because they are supposed to be. But not Patricia.

We protected her from some aspects of life, but we also tried to expose her to things she could use as she grew. We went places and did things that most other parents skipped. If it was local, sometimes we'd see other families there, but there weren't very many, and those who were there were usually the same ones: At the field at the elementary school watching the eclipse; or the Northern Lights that time they ventured down to Massachusetts for the first time in 20 years. Patricia spent the Millennium in Times Square. She met Mel "Today's the day" Fisher. We read. She read. She volunteered.

Music was a part of her life. She played the viola. She was good. Not great. But good. Her music teachers liked her. And she listened to other music too. But apparently not the kind real people listen to. I remember one day when she was about 10. I asked her what her favorite musical group was. She looked at me kind of funny. I asked again. She said it was when she got together with her friends and they played their instruments together. I was expecting the Back Street Boys.

∞

We were careful about what was on the TV. *Sesame Street* and The Discovery Channel. We went to lots of movies. Animated classics. Not the weird stuff.

My earliest recollection of bad parenting happened the day *Jurassic Park* came out on video. Patricia was in preschool. For some reason, I decided she was old enough to see her first real movie. The computer-generated creatures were incredible. And the story had all kinds of really cool science behind it. It also had gigantic dinosaurs eating the actors in one gulp. Somehow, I missed the fact that this was significant when I first saw it on the big screen. This was a bad idea. Very bad. Patricia didn't care for it at all. The next morning, I confessed my mistake to the preschool teacher and told her to call me if Patricia started screaming. *Sorry.*

Luckily, this didn't happen again until she was 13. Kate and I took her to see a movie called *Dus*. It's a Bollywood crime drama. Lots of guns. Lots of blood. Lots of death. I don't know what we were thinking. Patricia sat between us. I could hear her sobbing. I wasn't smart enough to walk out at the first shot. More bad parenting. Patricia still hasn't forgiven us for taking her. I don't blame her.

We saw two other important movies that year, *Thirteen* and *Paper Clips*.

Patricia was 11 when *Thirteen* came out. I always knew I wanted her to see it. It's a movie about a 13-year-old girl who experiences adolescence in a particularly negative way. There is shoplifting. Sex. Drugs. And deliberate self-injurious behavior: cutting. This movie is rated R. Here I had a real moral dilemma: Normally, R-rated movies are reserved for adults, but this was a story about the struggles of becoming an adult. If I waited until she was older, it would be too late. My goal has always been to give my children information. Let them see things they can use to make decisions for themselves as they mature. I decided we would watch it shortly after her 13th birthday. We did. It was brutal.

And we talked about it. *Do you have friends who take drugs?* "They aren't my friends." *Have you heard of cutting?* "Yes." *Do you know anyone who does?* "I think so." And I went on to tease her for a while longer. We'd been having conversations like this for years. Apparently, parents are supposed to do this. It's awkward.

I first heard about cutting as a contemporary problem when Patricia was in sixth grade, her first year of middle school. The principal, Dennis Easton, held a Coffee and Chat every month. These were legendary; stories about them had filtered down to the elementary school. Besides getting the principal's take on what was going on, there was another draw: He would answer any question posed by the audience. And, he would answer it honestly. For parents of middle school kids, this presents an opportunity for great entertainment. Groups of giggly mothers attended. They'd ask thoughtful questions. Ultimately, there usually weren't very many of us there. More often than not, I was the only father. He made me feel welcome.

For a couple of years, I tried to sit in the back and be inconspicuous. I was very quiet and didn't talk to anyone. I hoped he didn't know my name. Even more, I hoped he didn't associate me with Patricia. Kids have enough trouble growing up without being related to their parents. I had run into this same problem with PTA meetings at the elementary school. Apparently, parents who show up for these things do so because they want to help. To volunteer. To put their name down on the signup sheet to run the bake sale. Or the fall festival. Not me. I was there to listen. To see what was going on. To hover quietly in the background and make sure others weren't screwing up my kid. I was capable of doing that myself, thank you.

This worked. For a while. Until I started to hear things that didn't make sense. When I couldn't stand it anymore, I started asking my own questions. The ladies in the PTA never answered my questions; they only squirmed. Dennis Easton squirmed too. But then he smiled; and answered them. His meetings were great.

Dennis introduced us to the idea of cutting during the spring of Patricia's sixth grade year. He reported that some seventh graders had been cutting. This is where you take a pen, or a paper clip, or a razor, and cut yourself. To draw blood. Children do this, he explained, to relieve anxiety. To reduce tension. Sometimes you cut on the wrist. Or the forearm. Or the leg. It's messy. It makes for big, ugly scabs. It leaves scars. Children get caught, usually because of the scabs and scars. Or a friend tattles on them. After that, the cutting moves to more hidden places.

Remember how I said I was naïve? I'd never heard of this. Dennis went on to explain that girls do it more than boys. Seventh grade is a popular time to start. And the smart ones, the ones in the top 10%, are usually the most vulnerable. Apparently, it takes a lot of effort to become a high-achieving girl. This causes anxiety. High-achieving girls give the illusion of having it all together. This attracts other girls who also would like to have it all together. These other girls attach themselves to the high-achieving girl. Then they dump all of their problems and insecurities on the high-achieving girl. They expect answers. They expect solutions. This leaves the high-achieving girl, who is already beset with the anxiety associated with becoming a high-achieving girl in the first place, with the additional anxiety of feeling obligated to solve the problems of others. Even though she might not actually have all the answers herself.

This, according to Dennis, leads to cutting. And it usually happens when a small bunch of high-achieving girls get together and decide that the only way they can get some relief is to try this cutting business. Dennis said that one of the most popular ways to do it is while instant messaging on the computer. And it works. Cutting actually makes them feel better. It's not an intent to die, or a cry for help, it's just to get relief.

Patricia is not a high-achieving girl. She was in the 88th percentile. Safely out of the top 10. Patricia has access to a computer, but not to IM. Too dangerous. We'd learned that at a talk at the school. And keep the computer in a public place. Ours was in the kitchen. There was no way Patricia could be cutting in the kitchen while doing stuff on the computer. Safe there, too. Most importantly, I read to Patricia. I'd been doing it for years. Bath time was our designated reading time. You need one of those every day. Taking one just before bedtime seemed reasonable, so we read every night for thousands of nights while Patricia took a bath or a shower. As she grew up, we added shower curtains and tried to increase her privacy, but even when she was 11, there were still a couple of seconds every night as she wrapped up in her towel and stepped out of the tub when I could see her ankles, her forearms and her wrists. No cuts. My child is safe. *Whew.*

After a stressful day of seventh grade, Patricia started cutting. She was just 13. We hadn't seen the movie yet. We'd moved reading from the tub to the couch, so I'd lost my comforting confirmation that everything was OK. She didn't learn it from her friends. She figured it out herself. She did it alone. The night she admitted to me that she'd taken some pills and had cut, she said, "The pain of cutting makes the sadness go away." She was frightened by the sadness. She said, "I don't know what to do if it comes back." I could see the panic in her eyes. Thinking about it now, cutting seems like a perfectly reasonable response to what was actually going on with her. But it took me a while to get there, because it took me a long time to actually see her darkness.

Paper Clips is the other movie we saw when Patricia was 13. This is a documentary about what happened when one class's

Holocaust unit at Whitwell Middle School in rural Tennessee got a little out of control. They set out to collect six million paperclips to get a sense of what the number six million actually feels like. One paperclip was to represent the life of each Jew extinguished by Adolf Hitler. It remains one of the most powerful movies I have ever seen. Of course, I took my children to see it. I wanted them to see how life can go on even after abominable acts of cruelty. Unfortunately, this is a skill we all need to have.

Seeing this movie helped Patricia survive the foolhardy Holocaust unit she had later at her own school. It was the spring of eighth grade. Kate was busy relearning how to walk after her stroke. Patricia had already "taken some pills." I was still clueless. One evening, Patricia was sitting at the computer, sobbing. I asked her what was wrong. She said she was writing a poem, but it was stuck.

It turns out that I did know about this poem. Something called team teaching had been going on for a couple of weeks. It's all the rage in progressive middle schools. It's when the history teacher delegates the Holocaust unit to the language arts teacher. Every night, for way too many nights, Patricia and all her classmates were each writing a new poem, in a different style, about the Holocaust. This has got to be the stupidest idea anyone has ever come up with. But I hadn't had a chance to bring it up at Coffee and Chat yet. The problem is that there are two kinds of kids in middle school: Those who already know about the Holocaust. And those who need to write a new poem, every night, for way too many nights, about the Holocaust, so they can learn about it. Patricia already knew about the Holocaust. Writing each new poem became an exercise in finding a new way to describe something indescribable, every night, for too many nights.

Patricia was sobbing. There was a poem. Stuck. In her. We talked enough for me to understand the problem. I'm still not sure if I did the right thing, but I decided that the best solution was to get it out of her. Write it down. I suggested this. I could see the panic on her face. This is not something she wanted to do. I persisted. Here is what she wrote. It took her about one minute. It was already done. Stuck. Inside her. She handed it to me:

Boxes of macaroni
Of toys and spark plugs, too
But boxes aren't for people
This I thought you knew

Real boxes are similar
Each pencil is the same
You cannot box people
Each person has a name

Chris was Jewish, just like me
You made him wear a star
Just because of what he believed
You left him with a scar

Jess's faith was Jewish, too
But her hair, it was still blonde
After her torture she was in a coma
I couldn't make her respond

Jenny was Jewish also
My sister oh so dear
But she can no longer hear birdsongs
You hurt her in the ear

All my siblings were lucky
All three of them survived
Unfortunately, I'm dead now
No longer could I have thrived

And now my siblings are lost
Without their older sis
They're like sheep without their shepherd
Jenny, Jess, and Chris

You thought that we were all the same
Like manufactured clocks
Hitler, do you remember me
I'm the one from in the box

I read it. When she turned around, I burst into tears. I knew I had made a terrible mistake. I also knew that her middle school had made a far more serious one.

Patricia is the greatest. I couldn't imagine how a 13-year-old kid could write something like that after getting hammered for too many weeks of writing poetry about the Holocaust. I was so proud of her. I told her that. I made her promise me that she would include this poem somewhere in her first published work. She reluctantly agreed.

Patricia admitted to me later that she had cut again that night. She had stopped. She had been feeling better. But she needed to cut that night.

∞

Shortly after the poem fiasco was over, the Holocaust unit set out on their next disaster: The Holocaust Memorial Project. A diorama! Those are cool. I like dragging my family to see dioramas. I sometimes wonder why their smiles aren't as big as mine. Every student's task was to design a Holocaust memorial. Patricia had to build a small scale replica of her memorial, design the exhibits, specify where her memorial was to be built, and explain why.

Patricia's came together over the course of several days. She talked with me about it. She asked my permission to include some elements of the story I told her of my visit to New York City the weekend after September 11, 2001. I obliged, and she came up with something I still think that someone, perhaps she, actually needs to build. She designed a series of three kiosks—you know, those things they have in France and in shopping malls—a big round post with a bigger round roof. One kiosk was plastered with the names, pictures, and accomplishments of Jews and descendants of Jews who survived the Holocaust. The other two kiosks were plastered with missing posters, just like those covering every available square inch of New York City after September 11. They were the pictures and stories of people who Patricia invented: Jews and the descendants of Jews who didn't survive the Holocaust, and the accomplishments that never happened because they weren't there. "Missing: Uncle Ned, who cured cancer. Have you seen him?" People like that. The missing people got two kiosks. Because that's the percentage Hitler got. She decided her memorial should be placed along the exit walkway from the Children's Holocaust Memorial railcar outside Whitwell Middle School in Whitwell, Tennessee. That class had gotten themselves a German cattle car, one used to transport thousands of victims to their deaths at concentration camps, parked it next to their school, and filled it with 11 million paper clips. In addition to 6 million Jews, Hitler wiped out 5 million others.

After Patricia showed it to me and went away, I burst into tears again. I was so proud of her. We had exposed her to things as she was growing up. She understood the Holocaust. We were good parents after all. When Patricia brought it to school and explained it to her teacher, the teacher asked her what a kiosk was. Patricia came home mad.

It took me a while, but I did talk with Principal Easton about this. Not in public at a Coffee and Chat. But quietly in his office. I told him about the kiosk. I brought Patricia's poem for him to read. I did this because he needed to hear what was going inside my kid's head. Maybe so he could help protect the next child from the same fate. He listened. And I think he heard me. Three years later, as part of her own Holocaust unit, Beth watched the movie *Paper Clips* with her classmates. She came home from school that night and asked me if I would take her to Whitwell Middle School the next time I went to Tennessee. She wants to see the memorial. I intend to.

I decided that these stories were another important part of Patricia's history.

∞

So is suicide.

One cold and sad December 29th, 15-year-old Brian Sculthorpe took his own life. His father, Gregg, found him at home. Gregg's efforts to revive his son were unsuccessful.

Gregg was at our home two weeks earlier, the day Kate had her stroke. Three days after that, Patricia had "taken some pills," but no one knew that yet. Two years earlier, we had all spent a perfect week cruising to Bermuda. I remembered Brian as the happy, smiley kid. Just like my kids, but a little bit older.

His death was devastating.

Gregg made a decision right off. I will respect him forever for it. I knew it was something I could never do. Instead of sweeping it under the rug and calling it some tragic accident, our town got to experience a real teen suicide. We talked about it. We grieved. We talked about Brian and his tragic death. We talked about the finality of it.

A permanent solution to a temporary problem.

I was still in shock after Kate's stroke. I was just getting used to being mom and dad and bus driver for my children. Somehow, I managed to make it to both the calling hours and the funeral.

Calling hours were different. Usually there is some quiet conversation in the hall and in line. And little smiles. Not today. There was an eerie silence. Silent nods. Pictures of Brian stared at us as we waited in line. But unlike the funeral of someone who has experienced a more complete life, these pictures were of a smaller snapshot in time. These were pictures of times I remembered. His soccer ball was quiet. The Yankees hat he wore on the boat just sat there, lifeless, on the table. I offered my condolences to Gregg and his family. I never know what to say at things like this. I really should write something on the back of my hand. But at times like this, finding the right words may not be possible. If I had the time, and the guts, I might have said something like this:

> *I am so sorry for your loss. I know I can't imagine what you must be going through, but I do know it must be something I could never handle as well as you are doing today. I am so thankful that my child is not lying there. I wish yours didn't need to be either. It's so unfair.*

The funeral was different, too. I knew the rector who presided over the service. He has a couple of boys nearly Brian's age. Somehow, he helped us all celebrate the life of a wonderful person who left us under such tragic circumstances.

Permeating these events was something else that was different. Unusual. Children. Maybe we are supposed to call them young adults, but these were 15-year-old kids in a place where 15-year-olds don't belong. And while you could say that they acted like perfect little young adults, what I saw were perfect little kids saying goodbye to one of their own who had left us too soon. It's so unfair.

During these days, I saw something else happening. And it comforted me. Our town was coming together. It began to wrap its arms around Gregg and his family. Just like the town had begun to do for me and mine after Kate had her stroke two weeks earlier. They were doing the same thing, but in a much bigger way, for Gregg. I knew he would be OK, just like I was beginning to believe that we might be OK too. For now. I hope he can stay OK.

Usually, when something terrible happens, it goes away within a couple of days. Life moves on. We put the memories in a dark place and try to get on with the job of living in the light. Not so with Brian's death. Gregg chose to use this as a learning tool. A way to make meaning out of the life of his only child. There was a feature article in the newspaper. A picture of Gregg sitting in Brian's empty room. We got to know the good things about Brian, and we got to see his struggles. And we got to see that he put a great deal of effort into trying to do his best—even if he wasn't always successful. Talk of a scholarship began to circulate. One that would acknowledge the accomplishments of a student who struggled, but ultimately had begun to pull it together.

I decided that this was going to be a learning experience for my family too. I was shaken up by his death. I let it show. My family saw my pain. I talked with my children about Brian. We remembered him. They began to talk about him. This was my goal.

As with most things, my family doesn't act in a normal, predictable way. That's not our style. And it isn't as much fun. Instead, we look for some way to make it more memorable. I'm the instigator. Brian's death was not going to be the exception. Sure, we'd make a donation to his scholarship fund, but we needed to do something else, too. Somehow I knew that at least part of it needed to have something to do with reading. We talked about it for a couple of months. And it let Brian's memory stay with us. Beth would be entering middle school in the fall. I was beginning to look forward to reading my Middle School Trilogy aloud to her. These are three books I had read to Patricia during the summer before she entered sixth grade. They complement each other. And they begin to introduce more disturbing, worldly themes into our reading. The first book is *To Kill a Mockingbird*. Next is *Good Night, Mr. Tom*. Finally, *Tangerine*. The first is about society and its flaws. The second is about family and its flaws. *Tangerine* is about adolescence and its flaws. It's told through the eyes of a young soccer player who learns that trying to grow up can be tough. Although the story is different, I see some of Brian's struggles in him. Brian played soccer.

Somehow, I knew that we would remember Brian through the book *Tangerine*. We talked about it some more. And it let Brian's memory stay with us for a little while longer. Ultimately, we decided to release 50 copies of *Tangerine* to travel around the world, each with an inscription of some kind, including Brian's name, inside the front cover. We already knew how to start books around the world; we'd been doing it for years. And we knew how to track them. With the help of *www.BookCrossing.com*, you can register a book online, print out a label describing that this is a free book—one to read and pass along—or leave somewhere in public for others to find—and then hope the next reader is willing to journal its journey online using the unique ID number printed on the label. Before passing it along again. Something like *www.WheresGeorge.com*, except for books instead of dollar bills.

I also decided it was appropriate to make a contribution in Brian's name to the Kristin Brooks Hope Center. They are the people behind the technology that routes phone calls from 1-800-SUICIDE to local people who are prepared to do something. That was the number listed in the crisis section of our local phone book. I decided that the best way to make a difference in my hometown was to make it so the next person who was thinking about suicide would have a place to call for help. We talked about it. And it let Brian's memory stay with us. I mailed a check.

The books were more complicated. I knew I needed to talk with Gregg about it first. I needed his permission to inscribe Brian's name in the front of those books. When you Google Brian's name, you end up at a link to that feature article. The one with Gregg's picture. I needed to make sure he could handle it. I wondered if I could handle it. I wrote some notes. I picked up the phone a number of times. I chickened out. Finally, I made the call and arranged to meet with Gregg.

This is like calling hours, only worse, and five months late. Here you really do need to know what to say. All kinds of things aren't appropriate. I settled on this: "I've been thinking about what I can do—for me—for Brian." We met. He gave me permission to include Brian's name in my book project. Within a couple of days, Kate, Patricia, and Beth helped me pack up 50 books and start them on their journey. The inscription inside the front cover reads, "To remember Brian Sculthorpe of Holden, Massachusetts." The *BookCrossing.com* sticker leads them to an online journal entry that says, "It's tough being a kid." Because it is.

Some books went to my sister-in-law who was finishing up teaching for a year in Idaho. She promised to give some to her school and sprinkle the rest at Laundromats and truck stops along her car ride home to New Hampshire. Other books went to a school in Canada after a teacher there wondered why I had so many copies of the book registered at *BookCrossing.com*. She was thinking about reading it with her class. I told her Brian's story. I knew that some of her students would figure out the significance of the inscription. She said she understood. That it was OK. And that she'd had similar experiences in her life, too. Small world. Being a kid really is tough.

The day after the books left for Idaho was the day Patricia told me about "the pills." I am convinced that our conversations about Brian, remembering him as we did, played a big part in Patricia's decision to confide in me. And if it weren't for Gregg's decision to use Brian's death as a teaching tool, Patricia might not ever have had the strength to seek help. *Thank you, Gregg.*

The other thing Brian's story gave me was great comfort that Patricia would be safe. She had seen the pain his death had caused his family. She had seen what his death did to our family. She had experienced what his death did to her. She had participated, for months, in remembering Brian. I was convinced that because of this, Patricia would never make another suicide attempt.

It turns out that I was wrong.

Because suicide isn't logical.

I decided that Brian's story was another important part of Patricia's history.

∞

Our intake appointment with Mark Wilkins was scheduled and getting closer. I was working on my list of things that might be important: Mom's stroke, smart kid, contemplative, wise beyond her years, music, books, movies, Brian, Holocaust unit. But there must be more. Except for her time at home, she spent the rest of her life at school or with friends. Friends? What about them? Patricia had friends. Some of them were real. But others were imaginary.

When Patricia was younger, Kate was her walking-line lady on the way to elementary school. Patricia spent some of those days talking with others in line with her, but she spent just as much time walking with mom and telling her fanciful tales of her imaginary friends. She told stories of their times together having vicarious adventures. Kate and I always smiled knowingly, proud of our kid with the creative mind.

Patricia had several real friends, too. A couple of them were good ones. They didn't always tolerate each other, particularly when too many of them got together at once, but Patricia could spend pleasant times with each of them. Some of them even arranged a surprise party for her 13th birthday. I was the designated driver. It was my job to drop her off at her friend's house; they'd jump out from behind the trees, yell, "Surprise!" and have cake. I was a little nervous; if anyone ever did that to me, I'd have a cow. But Patricia was fine. She was very pleased. She told me it was nice to have friends who would do that for her. No problem there.

∞

Patricia was involved with Destination Imagination. DI is an international creative problem-solving program for kids. It's an amazing thing to experience. Fellow students, from kindergarten to college, form teams with anywhere from two to seven members. They select from one of several challenges to work on. And they meet. And they meet. For months. And months. And the result is an eight-minute school play, "solving the challenge," in an age-appropriate, creative way. 100% kid-generated. No adult interference. It's incredible.

Patricia started with DI when she was in third grade. I spent the first year sitting in the corner during the meetings. Sitting on my hands. Not interfering. Just observing. Just making sure it wouldn't screw up my kid. The next year, and for a few years after that, I managed Patricia's teams. It was a perfect fit for me. I got to sit on their side of the room; still sitting on my hands; not talking; not interfering. Patricia loved DI. She looked forward to every meeting.

Mostly.

Because.

Because children act childishly. It's in their nature. They haven't completely mastered the intricacies of society. Seven children on a DI team sometimes means seven kings. Or seven court jesters. Destination Imagination showed me something about Patricia I'd seen before, but couldn't quite articulate. Or need to.

Patricia would get nervous—anxious—when children acted like children. Not only was Patricia the perfect child, but she expected that all children around her would be perfect too. And she took it personally and handled it badly when other children weren't being respectful and focused. This presents a problem for a creative problem-solving program that is supposed to be driven by children: They drive. Patricia tenses up. They squabble. Patricia shuts down. They vote to extend snack for the rest of the meeting rather than working on their solution, and before you know it, Patricia is the one sitting in the corner. Sobbing.

∞

School seemed OK. She was getting great grades. More than any parent could wish for. Homework was manageable. She read everything, including most of her schoolbooks. She wasn't one of the high-achieving girls, but right up there where I wanted her.

However, the night Patricia told me about "the pills" and the sadness, she also told me she sometimes felt like the character Nora Rowley from Andrew Clements's book, *The Report Card*. I remembered Nora as an overachieving fifth-grader who is so uncomfortable with her own success that she purposefully does badly on her schoolwork in hopes that her classmates might think she is normal. *Uh-oh.*

This is a little like the fourth-grade geography bee. We got a note from Patricia's school saying she was one of the finalists and we could come watch the playoffs. Patricia looked a little nervous on stage, but she was doing great. She lasted until the final two. When Patricia ultimately came in second, she burst into tears. Her classmates concluded she was a sore loser. But Kate and I knew they were tears of joy—she was relieved she hadn't come in first. The thought of going on to compete in the town finals was more than Patricia could handle. Apparently, we had a competitive kid. Who wanted to do well. Just as long as she didn't win.

Maybe that was an important part of her history as well.

∞

In late July, we met with Mark Wilkins at his Gardner office. Patricia was sullen. He asked Patricia why she was here today. Patricia sobbed. I said that Patricia had admitted to me that she had taken some pills. *Oh. When did you take the pills?* "Last December." *How many?* "Fourteen." You know the drill. Patricia didn't say much. Most of the questions were directed at me: Kate's stroke, smart kid, contemplative, wise beyond her years, creative, music, books, movies, Brian, Holocaust unit, friends, Destination Imagination, sensitive, fragile, Nora Rowley.

And that her family was a little strange, but we were that way on purpose and had a good time being that way. "What about a family history of mental illness?" Huh? *Uh-oh.* Maybe. *We'll get back to you.* We checked. It turns out that there was—in both my family and in Kate's. *How come nobody told me?* Or, maybe they did, and I wasn't listening.

Patricia contracted for her safety with Mark. We left his office with a promise that someone would call within a couple of weeks to set up a first appointment with a psychotherapist. "What's a psychotherapist?" *Someone to talk to.*

This happens all the time. She'll be fine.

But I was wrong. Three days later, near midnight, as I was resting in my chair—my recliner—Patricia came downstairs.

Then, she told me. Again.

"Dad, I took some pills."

+ ⬡10 + ◖4 + ⬡10 + ◖4

First Hospitalization

Patricia seemed OK in the days after her appointment with Mark Wilkins. There was a great sense of relief in having made it through this meeting. We didn't use the "s" word, even once. Patricia was safe; she had contracted for it again. She seemed relieved. She seemed grateful that I'd finally been able to arrange this after so long. Dad, the greatest. I'd spoken up for Patricia when she couldn't and I'd said everything I needed to say. During my Quest, I hadn't found that one thing I wanted to find. But I was feeling hopeful. I was amazed at how much information I was able to assemble about Patricia's history in just two short weeks. I'd always been the aloof dad, but I liked that too. Apparently, I really had been paying attention to at least some things going on around me for all those years.

∞

Reading to the children was my one true passion. We'd been doing it for years. Nearly every night. When Patricia was little, I would read her *Goodnight Moon*, or *A Pocket for Corduroy*, or *The Poky Little Puppy*. Over and over. Night after night. For hundreds of nights. I always assumed that once Patricia learned to read, my job would be over. Patricia was pretty smart, so I was beginning to dread the day.

When Patricia was in nursery school, I went to a parent program at the local elementary school about family reading. Even though we already knew how to read, I decided to go anyway. And sit in the back. And listen. Just to make sure I hadn't been screwing up my kid. It turns out that reading aloud to your children is OK. *Good to know.*

I learned two more things that night: The first is that children's literature had changed since I was a kid. I sat there and listened to our town librarian talk passionately about books. Librarians are supposed to do that; it's their job. But what I was experiencing was more than that. This lady actually believed that books were interesting. And she gave us some examples: *Hatchet*, the story of another Brian's survival despite acts of unspeakable cruelty rained down on him by Mother Nature, and *Holes*, a new book about digging for clues to your own history. I had to read them.

The second thing I learned that night is you are allowed to continue to read to your child even after they've learned to read for themselves. No one does it, but it's allowed. The next day, I went to the bookstore, snuck into the children's section—a place where I had never been and where I thought fathers weren't even allowed—found the books I was looking for, brought them home, went into my closet, turned on my flashlight, and read them all. They were amazing. Things had changed since I was a kid. These books were actually interesting. They talked about real problems. Real issues. *Uh oh.* Patricia was four.

That's when I really started on my first Quest. I spent years searching for the perfect books to read to Patricia. We started with books that were a little calmer. Books I could read to her as we got ready to read the books I really wanted her to experience. And during that time, we found lots of great books. Books for younger kids. Books that dealt with younger kid issues. Eventually, I overcame my fear of bookstore clerks. And librarians. Since then, they have been a great source for ideas on important books to read to my children. I didn't realize until years later that, like firefighters, librarians and bookstore clerks have a passion in life: To help fathers find the next perfect book to read to their kid. Or at least the good ones do.

As we read, I overcame another fear: The idea that a book, particularly a chapter book, is just too big to read aloud to a kid. It turns out that if you read nearly every night, for years, you end up reading tens of thousands of pages. That's hundreds of books. The other thing reading did was put us together. I got to spend time—about 40 minutes each day—one on one—reading to each kid. I was never a good conversationalist, and I certainly didn't know how to talk with children, but reading passed the time, and for a few minutes each day, at the beginning or the end of our story, we'd talk. About little things. About problems and worries. It made it so I really did know about some of the things going on in my children's lives. And it made me accessible. I could talk to them. And they could talk to me.

In the time before our appointment with Mark Wilkins, Patricia and I talked. We did it in quiet little pieces, just like we had for years as we read together. It made it possible for me to fill in some of the blanks as I was trying to put together her history for The Quest. It also gave me hope because she appeared to be open and honest about how she was feeling, something that I did know is not a normal characteristic of adolescence. I was proud of her. My daughter, who "took some pills." Years later, I credit her honesty with keeping her alive through some very difficult times.

∞

For a couple of nights after our meeting with Mark Wilkins, Patricia didn't go to bed. This was unusual. The perfect child was always in bed at a reasonable hour. We had a rule that said you must be in bed on time, but you could read for as long as you wanted. I go to bed very late, and it wasn't unusual for Patricia to still be awake when I walked by her room on my way to bed. At one a.m. Or two. I'd tease her about it. But she was always in bed. That night, and the next night, she came back downstairs after getting into her pajamas and we watched movies together until three. I didn't push it. It just seemed like the right thing to do.

The next night she had a babysitting gig. Although she had agreed to spend some time with me when she got home, she went right upstairs to bed. *Good. Back to normal. Everything will be fine.*

The following afternoon, Patricia took the dog for a long walk. Very long. After an uneventful evening, by 11 p.m., she was still wandering around the house. Patricia commented that the frogs had been out earlier, so we decided to go out on an adventure. Once a year, some years, when the planets and the stars line up just right, a mass frog migration occurs on the streets of our town. Thousands or millions of small frogs, about the size of a small frog, decide they need to be elsewhere. So they go elsewhere. The immediate result is that the streets are covered with frogs. All hopping madly from one side to the other. Some one way, some the other. And there are lots of them. Enough that you have to watch out to avoid stepping on them.

The secondary result, because some of our roads are actually used by cars—in addition to frogs—is that the thousands or millions of frogs, hopping madly from here to there, are doing it among the squished remains of thousands or millions of their brethren whose night of frivolity was cut short by one of those cars, on a trip to market to buy milk. It was gross. We walked the neighborhood. Trying to appreciate the incredible sight we were witnessing, all the while trying to ignore the carnage all around us.

We talked. Quietly. Carefully stepping around the issue. Patricia mentioned again how she felt like Nora Rowley, the character in that book. I didn't know what this meant. I didn't know how to help her.

When we came home, we read. It was her idea. She brought a book over, handed it me, and sat down to listen. We read for a while, and then she went upstairs to take a shower.

Near midnight, Patricia made another suicide attempt. She swallowed 40 Motrin pills. One minute later, she came downstairs and told me. *When?* "Just now." *What?* "These." She showed me the bottle. *How many?* "Forty."

This is about as far from the happy place I was in—sitting there in my recliner—as you can get.

Action!

Calling 911 was on the list. But not quite yet. I ran upstairs and told Kate. My immediate goal was to get those pills out of her stomach. Doing so turned out to be a challenge. Even with the help of my far-smarter-than-I-am wife. "Don't we have some syrup of pectate [sic]?" I asked. *That's syrup of ipecac, (dear,) and no, we don't have any.* The American Academy of Pediatrics had recommended getting rid of all the syrup of ipecac in America's medicine cabinets, and of course my wife was watching TV that day. So there wasn't any.

The Internet wasn't any help. Even if we had a computer and data connection as fast as the fastest supercomputer at the National Security Agency, it still would have been too slow. When your child is dying of a drug overdose, nothing could ever be fast enough. I had to use my wits. And my wife's. My idea was to make her drink some baking soda and water. It didn't work. Kate's idea was to make her swallow a raw egg. That didn't work either. Patricia was not pleased with either idea, but she complied.

Next on the list was the poison control hotline. But they'd probably just tell me to call 911. So why didn't I just do that? It was easy. But the reason was that it would have delayed getting those pills out of my kid. They'd be quick, but it would take some time. "What happened?" *She took some pills.* "Why?" *I don't know.* You know the routine. By that time, those pills would be dissolved, and the only choice they'd have is to take her to the hospital. Because my perfect child had just "taken some pills."

We drove. Simple as that. Get into the car and drive to the hospital. A little fast and a little quick out of the stop signs, but safely and in control. We parked in the garage. And walked into the emergency room at about 12:15 a.m. Those pills had been in her for 17 minutes. At triage: *My daughter took some pills.* "What kind?" *These.* "How many?" *Forty.* "When?" *About 11:58.* "How did you find out?" *She told me.* Turning to Patricia, the nurse asked, "Why did you take them?"

"I don't know."

Everyone except me remained surprisingly calm. I just tried to maintain the illusion of calm. I was expecting teams of doctors descending on my child. Pumps. Hoses. Controlled vomiting. Kind of like in *Almost Famous*, another one of those films you need to see before you are ready for it, because if you wait too long, it will be too late. We hadn't seen it. Instead, the nurse came in with a paper cup and told Patricia to drink it. C&C. Except with a spoon in it instead of ice. Coke and charcoal. Thick and lumpy. I could tell from her face that it didn't taste like a smoothie. She nursed it for a long time: every time the nurse came in, she'd take another sip.

We'd been to the emergency room before. Stitches. Asthma, stuff like that. We had experience waiting. But this was a new kind of wait. We made it through triage in five seconds. A record. We had our own room in the ER. A nurse now and then. The charcoal. A doctor. Vital signs. A blood draw. A urine sample. Each one of which seemed to be separated by two hours of nothing. After what seemed like an eternity, a man arrived on the unit. He was dressed in khakis and a button down shirt with thin, pastel-colored, vertical strips. This guy just oozed psychologist, a term I knew I should know, but which hadn't yet made it into my lexicon. After what seemed like another two hours, he came over, introduced himself, and said, "I'm here to do an evaluation."

We determined the facts. There were lots of questions. Patricia answered them as best she could. She did a better job than she had three days earlier with Mark Wilkins. But there was really only one question that mattered, "Were you trying to kill yourself when you took those pills?"

"Yes." Another involuntary exhale from me.

He got up to leave, and as he did, he asked me a question, "Why did you come here? To this hospital, West Side?" Huh? I explained that there really wasn't any question about where to go. This was the closest hospital to our home. It was where Patricia was born, and it was the hospital we've been patronizing now and then over the years to sew up the mementos of growing up. It seemed like the right place to go.

It turns out that for hospitals, there are additional selection criteria besides location and reading material in the waiting room. Particularly when the answer to the question about whether you were trying to kill yourself is, "Yes." In addition to saving your life, there are a whole series of new issues that come up. Questions like, "If I let you go home, are you going to try it again?" It takes a special kind of doctor to ask these questions, and they don't work at West Side Hospital. They work at East Side Health Center, the other affiliated hospital just over the hill. No one ever told me that if your child "takes some pills," go to East Side Health rather than West Side Hospital. And we suffered for this. Even more than we were already suffering.

Pastel-stripe-guy needed to commute up and over the hill several times that night to visit with us at the wrong hospital. He went away. For a lot longer than it would have taken even me to walk up and over the hill and back. When he returned, he spoke with me. But first, he gave me a look. One I haven't seen since. I think now that it was empathy. He knew I was starting on something serious. Something frightening. Something over which I might not have complete control. I appreciated it. He asked me questions. I answered them as best I could. I had some notes from my Quest with me in my pocket, and I dragged them out. There were lots of pages: Kate's stroke, smart kid, contemplative, wise beyond her years, creative, music, books, movies, Brian, Holocaust unit, friends, Destination Imagination, sensitive, fragile, Nora Rowley, interesting family. He was patient. He asked about family history. I told him what I knew. As he was finishing up, he asked me one final question. But he prefaced it with a statement. He said, "I've already made my decision, but do you think Patricia will be safe if you take her home?"

Trick questions should not be allowed in hospitals. They should not be asked of stressed out fathers at six a.m. after a night of no sleep. And they should not be allowed in any circumstances when they are being asked by a doctor, a specialist whose specialty you never even knew existed until a few minutes (or hours) ago, particularly when the specialist already knows the answer to his own question. This isn't fair.

I said, "Yes."

He said, "No."

I agreed with him instantly.

Six hours later, Patricia was admitted to the Children's Psychiatric Unit at Patriot Medical Center in Wellesley, Massachusetts. Apparently, things move just as slowly, even if you have a plan. It's 25 miles from hospital to hospital. I followed behind the ambulance in my car. And it's 38 miles back to my house. I was home by one in the afternoon.

I slept for an hour, grabbed some things for Patricia, and drove the 38 miles back to Wellesley and the Children's Psychiatric Unit. An inconspicuous ward off a dark hallway. With a buzzer. Next to a locked door. With a tiny little window. Whose glass is reinforced with wire mesh. A mental hospital. For children.

Patricia spent 10 days there.

∞

Imagine being on vacation with your family in New York City. It's 7:59 p.m. and you're walking up Broadway. You've come across a busy theatre with a bright and glittery marquee: *Mental Health, the Musical*. A few of the lights are burned out. Obviously, this show has been running for a while now. But you've never seen it; you've heard of it, but beyond that, you don't know anything about it. As you pass the stage door, it opens. A shadow beckons you inside, and for some reason, you go in, family in tow. You find yourself on a darkened stage. You can sense that there are other people onstage and in the audience, but it's too dark to see who or how many are there. Suddenly, the lights come up, and you find that you and your whole family have just become the stars of one of the longest running shows in theatrical history.

Except you have no talent. And you're a little shy. And you don't know any of the words.

The other actors around you burst into song. They sound like they've done this before. Your only job is to carry the show.

∞

Dr. Chase was our contact at Patriot Medical. He said that he was the psychologist. He introduced us to the hospital's child psychiatrist. I wondered which one of them might be that psychotherapist thing we'd been trying to get Patricia hooked up with for the past two months. This was starting to get complicated. Dr. Chase went on to tell us that the social worker was on maternity leave, he was doing her job, too, so Patricia would only be getting half the services she was entitled to receive. I didn't know whether I should be concentrating on the only getting half the services part, whatever that meant, or this new word, "social worker."

Dr. Chase said that the average stay on the ward was four days. Their goal was to stabilize Patricia and send her home into the care of an outpatient psychiatrist and a psychologist. We've already established that I don't know what those are, but it was still my job to find them and schedule appointments. In the meantime, Patricia would bunk in one of the rooms, probably with a roommate near her age. She would be attending groups, but because this was summer, school wasn't necessary. Things would begin in earnest on Monday when most of the staff returned, except, of course, for the social worker. In addition to all the staff whose names begins with "psy," we met the head nurse, some of the weekend nursing staff, and a couple of counselors. Just like camp. They all sang their parts beautifully.

Patricia met with the psychiatrist later in the day. They began what would turn out to be another Quest. One to find the right combination of medicines to give Patricia some relief. She started on Prozac, for depression, and another drug, Trazodone, to help with anxiety.

That night, Patricia slept for perhaps the first time in her life. She commented on it the next day. Sleep. Real sleep. And she fell right to sleep. She slept through the night. She woke up refreshed and relaxed. This is not the report I was expecting from my child's first night in the mental hospital. The other kids were OK. And the staff was helpful when they needed to be. I was surprised how natural it felt to sit at the end of her bed, with her sitting next to me, and just talk. Quietly. About little things. As we had done thousands of times.

Safe.

Patricia was safe. But what about the rest of us? After driving home that afternoon, leaving one child in the warm embrace of the mental hospital, Kate, Beth, and I were visited by a summer storm. The technical term is derecho, but no one knows what that means. Think thunderstorm. Think microburst. Think destruction. After the skies darkened and took on that green tinge that usually foreshadows something exciting, the wind picked up. And it started to rain. When the lightening started, it didn't begin to the west, as usual. It was everywhere. The trees lit up and revealed a scene reminiscent of a Dr. Seuss book. The pine trees were bending in ways that seemed impossible. But the hundred-year-old oak in the front yard was doing something even more spectacular. It only took a couple of seconds, but that tree did a little dance. Followed by a curtsey. When it was all over, the front yard had been rearranged. The only thing standing was the bottom 15 feet of oak tree. Everything else was on the ground. On top of the electrical wires that formerly powered our home. When the lightening finally stopped, everything went black.

So while we sat at home in the dark, Patricia did a great job of integrating herself into the hospital routine. "Milieu" was the new word. It's a fancy term for mental hospital and the social environment associated with it. Kind of like the script of a Broadway play, except it includes the props and actors, too. There were patient rooms, a nurse's station, a community room, an art room, a classroom, a number of offices, an outdoor exercise yard—

just a boxed-in light shaft in the center of the building with high wire mesh walls—and a quiet room. The quiet room was the only space that matched my perception of what I was expecting: padded walls, a rugged door, one bed bolted to the floor, and armored lights and TV camera safely out of the way on the ceiling. The art room surprised me in its own way. It looked like a place where Jackson Pollock could have thrived when he was eight; or thirty-eight. There was paint dripped everywhere and every kind of art supply you could imagine. The rest of the place looked just like a hospital, with one difference: except for the patient rooms, every door was locked up tight.

By Monday, I started making telephone calls. I needed to find a psychiatrist and psychologist. I called Mark Wilkins's office and left a message.

No one called me back.

I met with Dr. Chase a number of times. It turned out I had a couple more jobs: making the house safe for Patricia's return home and learning new ways to interact with my child. We talked about "Dialectical Dilemmas: Finding the Middle Path – Balance." He had handouts from a skills training manual for suicidal adolescents, something adapted from Marsha Linehan's *Skills Training Manual for Treating Borderline Personality Disorder*. The first two handouts had to do with trying to find the balance between being too loose or too strict on parental rules and the importance that they be clear and consistently enforced. That the balance be found between making light of problem behaviors and making too much of adolescents acting like normal adolescents. The last handout had to do with the parents holding on too tight or forcing independence. Apparently, the answers to these questions matter, and how well the parent's answers align with the child's answers matters too. *Uh-oh.* My bad-parenting alarms were going off.

By this time, I'd been through my Patricia spiel with Dr. Chase: Mom's stroke, smart kid, and so on. But more than anything, great kid; more than you could ever want. We didn't have rules because we had the perfect kid. You asked, she did, simple as that. There weren't any problem behaviors—except perhaps for "taking some pills"—so we hadn't spent any time enforcing rules or making light of adolescent behaviors. We'd tried to give Patricia her independence, but we also wanted her to know we'd be available if she needed us. It had served us pretty well—except perhaps for the part about her "taking some pills." We did not resolve the dialectical dilemma that day. Or the next.

As the days passed, I spent a lot of time in the car driving back and forth to the hospital. It gave me time to think. One problem was finding those "psy" people. Mark Wilkins had called me back. He said that in light of "current circumstances" (I believe a code word for Patricia's new suicide attempt), Mark felt Patricia would be better served by a larger agency. One that had more staff and 24-hour coverage. He gave me some names. I left messages.

No one called me back.

The rest of my car time was spent working on this other impossible task: making our home safe for Patricia's return. For different kids, this means different things. For us, it meant locking up all the medicines. This was going to be difficult. I had a wife taking a boatload of stroke meds every day and two children who were on seemingly hundreds of allergy and asthma drugs. The medicine cabinets, both upstairs and down, were bursting with stuff. We had drawers of refills. We had every kind of pain pill in all those places and in every pocketbook and car. *Uh-oh.*

I lamented to the nurse about this. What did other families do? She suggested I find a locking medicine cabinet. *Where?* Actually, these do exist. I found some. Eventually. There are issues with stud spacing and other technical problems with swapping this out for one of our existing ones. But the biggest problem was this: they all needed a key. I knew that Patricia was the most reliable person in our house, and eventually, it would become her job to be the one who kept the key. The rest of us would lose it. This was not going to work. I was impressed by Patriot Medical's Parent Handbook. Lots of multicolored pages carefully indexed with everything rookie families needed to know. Why wasn't there a page on locking medicine cabinets? It was part of the script. It should have been there. But it wasn't.

This became a big problem. It lingered for a number of days, just like my child was lingering in the hospital longer than those four days we were expecting. Finally, Sears solved my problem.

Next to the hardware section are the safes, including rugged lockboxes with an electronic keypad on the front. I chose a good sized one and brought it home. We picked a combination Patricia wouldn't know and that we could remember. Medicines went inside. Some of them fit. The next day, I went back and bought the bigger one. Our house full of medicines comfortably filled both of them. As long as Patricia didn't need too many pills, we'd be fine.

The hospital psychiatrist doubled her medicines.

Finding a psychiatrist and psychologist for after the hospital was going badly. Dr. Chase kept asking how I was doing. Lousy. I was still waiting for a number of people to call me back. In desperation, I called Dr. Fitzgerald. When I'd called her to let her know Patricia had been admitted to Patriot Medical, she told me to call again if I ever needed something. Until now, I didn't know what to ask for. I made the call. She said she'd do some research.

A few minutes later, she called me back.

Did you hear that? She called me back. She said she would make a referral to the Massachusetts Child Psychiatric Access Project (MCPAP). It was a new program she'd just learned about. It matches children in Massachusetts with psychiatric professionals when an "emergency" (perhaps a code word for "taking some pills") comes up and there is trouble finding help. I was beginning to believe that another pattern was developing, one where there is always trouble finding help. Dr. Fitzgerald told me to expect a phone call from a social worker. That name again—social worker. Maybe time for more research.

Within a day, I did get a call from an MCPAP social worker. I told her the situation. About my calls. That I was waiting to hear from a number of people. She listened. She told me to call her back if I had trouble finding someone. We hung up. After I put the phone down, I picked it back up. To see if she was still there. Because we were having trouble finding someone. That's why I called. But there was only a dial tone.

∞

Things were getting serious. My kid was in the hospital. Progress toward coming home had stopped. It was time to talk with my family. There were a couple of reasons for this. One was that

Patricia wasn't at home; someone would figure it out and start asking questions. The more important one was that I needed help and I didn't know who else to call. I suspected my sister might have some experience with this, either in her own family, or through her job as a school psy-something-ist. I called her. She was very understanding. She listened to my tale of woe. She told me to call my insurance company and demand to talk with a supervisor. I did. It worked. I ended up speaking with a case manager. She listened. And then she told me it was the hospital's job to find outpatient providers and make appointments for when Patricia left the hospital. This was not my problem. The hospital should know that. Shame on them. When I told Dr. Chase this, he said, "Oh yeah. It is my job. But you should keep looking." I kept calling.

No one called me back.

After 10 days, Patricia was discharged home. Apparently, *Mental Health, the Musical* only has enough material for about six days. After that, it just repeats again from the beginning. New characters join the show every day or two, so your starring roles go to someone else and your family gets relegated to the chorus, but you are still there, on stage, performing every minute of every day. The problem is that if you aren't better after six days, the hospital doesn't know what to do. They told me Patricia was stable, even though I still didn't know what that meant.

But I did know that stable is different from better.

She had developed a Safety Plan. It's like a Contract for Safety, except written and more detailed. It lists a series of feelings, from OK to anxious, to need to cut, to suicidal ideation, to suicide. Next to each is an action step to feel better and remain safe: take a shower, walk the dog, talk to a trusted adult. It looked pretty good to me. They were pleased.

Dr. Chase found us a psychiatrist and a psychologist. He made appointments for the next day. It really was his job, after all.

Patricia came home. She slept in her own bed.

We filled the prescriptions for her new medicines and jammed them into the new lockboxes. We had a new regimen. Up at a reasonable hour. Medicines at 7:30 p.m., just like the hospital told us, then to bed at 9 p.m., 90 minutes later. Lather. Rinse. Repeat.

Patricia now had a mental health diagnosis. It is:
Depressive Disorder, NOS
Rule Out Anxiety Disorder.

"NOS" means "Not Otherwise Specified." We'll talk about that later. I still don't know what "Rule Out" means. I looked it up once. It didn't make any sense. And apparently some people use it to mean one thing and others think it means the exact opposite. I'll do some more research and we'll get back to that too.

(93 43) (433)

$$+ \text{\small(433)} + \text{\small(PD)} - \text{\small(434)} - \text{\small(PD)} + \text{\small(S193)} - \text{\small(S193)} + \text{\small(434)}$$

Side-Effects

The next morning, we went to Lee Street Family Services, a clinic in Worcester. We met with Richard, the director. He said he was a licensed social worker. He'd be doing the intake; and then we'd meet with his psychiatrist in the next room after lunch. Richard would select one of his many therapists for Patricia based on what he learned today. We went through the spiel again: Kate's stroke, smart kid, contemplative, wise beyond her years, creative, music, books, movies, Brian, Holocaust unit, friends, Destination Imagination, sensitive, fragile, Nora Rowley, interesting family. Every time I went through this, it took forever, but I had no idea what was important. When their eyes started to glaze over, I'd speak faster. When that didn't help, I'd start leaving things out. But hopefully, just the stuff that didn't matter. Whatever that was.

That afternoon, we met with the psychiatrist. We shook hands. We sat down. He began by clarifying that he was working for Lee Street Family Services today. He had another practice in Worcester, his name and number were in the phone book, but under no circumstances were we to ever phone him there. All contact must be made through Lee Street Family Services. Period. He worked here once a month. Patricia would need to make an appointment to see him on that day. His schedule was tight, so we might have trouble finding a time outside of school hours.

We talked, but in an abrupt and much more abbreviated way. Once again, Patricia didn't say much. Most of the questions were directed at me. Our chief complaint was about sleep. Unlike the first few days of glorious sleep in the hospital, it was getting harder to get to sleep. Patricia would take her medicines at 7:30. Thirty-five minutes later, she'd have this incredible wave of tiredness rush over her. She'd spend the next 55 minutes dragging herself around the house. When she actually went to bed, she couldn't get to sleep. It was frustrating.

He doubled the Trazodone. He stood. We shook hands. He said he was going on vacation. See you in September. Any problems, call the clinic.

We went home.

∞

August was a busy month. We had a kid, fresh home from the mental hospital, who wasn't sleeping. The hospital had warned us to be aware of Patricia's mood. She was on Prozac, an SSRI, a selective serotonin reuptake inhibitor. It's a kind of antidepressant. It comes with a black box warning on the label, just like cigarettes:

SSRI Black Box Warning

WARNING: Antidepressant medications are used to treat a variety of conditions, including depression and other mental/mood disorders. These medications can help prevent suicidal thoughts/attempts and provide other important benefits. However, studies have shown that a small number of people (especially people younger than 25) who take antidepressants for any condition may experience worsening depression, other mental/mood symptoms, or suicidal thoughts/attempts. Therefore, it is very important to talk with the doctor about the risks and benefits of antidepressant medication (especially for people younger than 25), even if treatment is not for a mental/mood condition. Tell the doctor immediately if you notice worsening depression/other psychiatric conditions, unusual behavior changes (including possible suicidal thoughts/attempts), or other mental/mood changes (including new/worsening anxiety, panic attacks, trouble sleeping, irritability, hostile/angry feelings, impulsive actions, severe restlessness, very rapid speech). Be especially watchful for these symptoms when a new antidepressant is started or when the dose is changed.

Huh? Why would you give a suicidal kid a drug that makes you more suicidal? This makes zero sense. There was even a handy checklist included with the prescription so we could play along at home. Here is the list:

SSRI Side-Effect Checklist

- ☐ *Thoughts about suicide or dying.*
- ☐ *Attempts to commit suicide.*
- ☐ *New or worse depression.*
- ☐ *New or worse anxiety.*
- ☐ *Feeling very agitated or restless.*
- ☐ *Panic attacks.*
- ☐ *Difficulty sleeping.*
- ☐ *New or worsening irritability.*
- ☐ *Acting aggressive, being angry, or violent.*
- ☐ *Acting on dangerous impulses.*
- ☐ *An extreme increase in activity and talking.*
- ☐ *Other unusual changes in behavior or mood.*

We spent the month of August checking things off the list. All but one: The one where she actually kills herself. Many got checked off on the first day. The others were added one by one as the weeks passed. Notice the part on the black box warning about telling your doctor right away if there are "unusual behavior changes …" We lived those every day. The receptionist at the clinic took my calls, but we never heard back from the psychiatrist or anyone who was covering for him during his vacation. If there was such a person.

In August, Patricia started seeing her new therapist, Debra White. She was wonderful. Patricia took to her and they met nearly every week for three years. They talked about everything. Some things I heard about; most I'll never know. More often than not, Patricia would come out of those sessions feeling better. Safe. Refreshed. Usually. On those days when she didn't, Deb would talk with me about what's going on with Patricia today. Most often, I already knew something was up. I was comforted that Patricia was sharing her feelings with Deb. Someone other than Patricia and me needed to know what was going on. Because someone needed to know when it was time to react. And what kind of reaction to make.

∞

We had a new problem. We were scheduled to go on vacation the last week in August. A cruise. To the Caribbean. This one was just our family. No other friends this time. We mentioned this to each new provider: Mark Wilkins, Dr. Chase, the clinic director, his now-missing psychiatrist, and Deb. We asked for their advice. To a person, they all recommended we keep our plans and go on vacation. They predicted that Patricia would have a great time.

After a couple of weeks, I met with the clinic director again. I expressed my frustration in being unable to get some feedback from his psychiatrist about these new symptoms. Even Deb was getting worried. He told me that his guy wasn't really the best choice for Patricia, but he was all he could find. He recommended we contact Raymond Counseling, a larger practice in Worcester. They had doctors. I called. They called back. We made an appointment for after our cruise.

The day before the cruise, I called Lee Street Family Services again. I told the receptionist I really needed to talk with the covering doctor. Patricia wasn't sleeping and I was concerned I wouldn't be able to get her to sleep on the boat. I was already sleeping on the floor next to her bed so she'd step on me if she got up in the middle of the night. I used my new concerned-father voice with the receptionist—the one I'd been practicing with all my free time—the one that's supposed to sound like I really need an answer and not just lip service. She promised to see what she could do.

A couple of hours later, she called me back. She asked if I had ever tried Benadryl for sleep. I said, "No." She told me to ask my pharmacist about it. This was ridiculous. Worse yet, I became a part of it. Here I was at the pharmacy signing up to have one of those private chats with the pharmacist. This wasn't something I wanted to discuss in public, so I was looking forward to having it in that room behind the new smoked-glass door labeled "Consultation Room." They're all the rage at the pharmacies near me. I guess they must eat their lunches in there, or store the photocopy paper, because we didn't have our consultation in there. We shouted it over the row of condoms and insulin supplies that separate us common folk from the pharmaceutical professionals. I told her about how the receptionist at my daughter's psychiatrist recommended Benadryl for sleep. She looked at me funny. I asked if she had any advice. She looked at me again. Then she told me to read the instructions on the box.

So off we went to the Caribbean with a box of Benadryl. In case Patricia couldn't sleep.

The cruise was a disaster.

As we walked on board, Patricia kept looking everywhere. Her eyes scanned the ceilings. When we walked by something, Patricia asked me if that was a camera. I said, "Maybe." "Probably." Patricia kept looking. It went on like that all the way to our cabin. I decided I wouldn't talk Patricia out of believing the ship was covered with cameras. I knew that some were. Most weren't. But it comforted me to know that Patricia thought there were cameras everywhere, with an army of security personnel watching the live feed, and that if she tried anything, "they" would stop her. By the time we got home, I was pretty sure this was the only reason Patricia didn't jump off the boat.

We'd been on cruises before. After a couple of days into the first one, you become "seasoned passengers." You learn the routine. Like Disney, they try very hard to make it easy to have a good time. That's the only reason people go back. We'd had children before, too. In fact, we'd actually cruised with these exact same ones. And they had always tried very hard to make it easy for us to be parents, and that was the only reason we ever brought them anywhere. But this time, something was different.

Patricia was now 14. Old enough to be with the older group of kids on the boat. Away from her sister, Beth. More freedom. No parental drop offs or signing in and out. Just dances. Scavenger hunts. Hanging out with other kids, hopefully just drinking soda. Patricia had always been able to make friends. But something was broken. "New or worse anxiety," number four on our handy checklist. "Panic attacks," number six. Because she'd done it before and knew how to have fun, her inclination was to go. But when it came right down to showing up, I could see the panic level rise in her. When she asked, I'd go along and wait outside. Other times, she wanted to go places on her own. I let her, but I worried.

Our cell phones, like most, didn't work at sea. We had family radios. Walkie-talkies. They had a signal in most places on the boat, so there was a bit of a sense of connectedness. But having a radio is not the same thing as being there when you are on a big giant ship in the middle of nowhere in the middle of a gigantic ocean. Patricia came back from her adventures with a look of relief more than one of contented satisfaction. One night, one of her new friends, parents in tow, delivered Patricia to our cabin a few minutes earlier than we were expecting her back. I could see some of that same look of relief on their faces as I opened the door. They were clearly scared by what they saw in Patricia. I thanked them. We talked quietly about anxiety. They seemed satisfied and left.

We made it home. Now I was the one who was relieved.

∞

School was starting in a couple of days. She would be a freshman at Abenaki Regional High School, one of the largest schools in Massachusetts. Patricia had never had trouble with school before, but if August was any indication, September was going to be a new experience for all of us. The day before school started, I made a decision. Just me. I didn't think about it for very long. And Patricia didn't get a vote or veto power, something I might have been inclined to offer in the past. I called up Brenda Harris, Patricia's new guidance counselor at Abenaki High and asked if we could come down and say hello. *Today.* She said, "Sure." So we went.

Introductions were made. Patricia actually spoke. They made small talk about the nervous anticipation of starting school tomorrow. I joined the conversation and added the words "depressed" and "safety plan." It was very clear to me that Brenda knew what was going on and had heard it all before. We left with new knowledge and a significantly reduced anxiety level. Patricia now knew where the guidance office was and that a friendly face would be there. Just in case. That visit made my phone call to her the next week that much easier.

On the afternoon of the first day of school, we met with Carol Sherman, a nurse practitioner at Raymond Counseling, to talk about Patricia's medicine. She was wonderful. She was the first person to actually talk directly to Patricia. She asked questions. Patricia answered them. Carol asked new questions, ones based on the answers Patricia had already given. I was hearing things from Patricia I didn't know to ask during my Quest. It was refreshing.

We had told the "Getting to Sleep" story to several people. The one where Patricia took her nighttime medicines 90 minutes before bedtime, she got very tired 35 minutes later, but once in bed, couldn't get to sleep. Carol said the wave of tiredness is the hint it's time to go to bed. Go to sleep then. If you miss it, you've got to figure out how to get to sleep on your own. Patricia had been having trouble with that for 14 years. Maybe we should let the meds help.

During this whole episode, Carol was very kind. She didn't snicker or pat me on the back of the hand or give me a funny look. I kind of wish she did, because I probably deserved it. Of course you go to bed when you are tired. Why wouldn't you? We had been trying so hard to follow the hospital's instructions. But we were ignoring reason. *Ugh.*

Carol replaced the Trazodone with Lunesta, a sleeping pill, to help with the bedtime routine.

Buried in each new prescription printout from the pharmacy is a list of possible side-effects. One of Lunesta's is "unpleasant taste." Of all the things that could go wrong—remember the list from Prozac—unpleasant taste doesn't sound too bad. Except: it was early September. Global warming was particularly bad that week, so the temperature was unseasonably high. Massachusetts schools aren't air conditioned. And the way this side-effect manifested itself with Patricia was that anything wet tasted like tinfoil—a metallic taste. Over the next two days, we learned about all kinds of wet things: juice, milk, watermelon, strawberries, water, and every other drink or food we tried to use to hydrate the kid. We also learned that given a choice between drinking tinfoil and nothing, Patricia chose nothing. Hands down.

Late on Friday afternoon, I reached a covering doctor at Raymond Counseling who stopped the Lunesta and restarted the Trazodone.

The metallic taste went away. But not before exhaustion and dehydration tossed a monkey-wrench into Patricia's life at her new high school. Things only got worse over the weekend. Patricia decompensated. Another new word. It's like being terrible, then being even more terrible, right before you are really terrible. On

Sunday, Patricia took the family dog for a walk. Not unusual, but a really long walk. When she got home, she told me that if she hadn't had mom's cell phone with her, she might have just walked forever rather than come home. When I asked what mom's cell phone had to do with it, she replied that "they" could track her with it. Later, when a doctor asked Patricia why she didn't just drop the phone on the ground and go, Patricia said it was mom's phone and that she was responsible for bringing it home. That was the day logic and reason left our lives. And when I started ruminating about how long forever might be.

93 43   434

$$+ \boxed{93\ 43} - \boxed{93\ 43} \boxed{93\ 43} - \bigodot{434} + \boxed{54\ 213} + \bigodot{100}$$
$$+ \boxed{54\ 213} + \boxed{54\ 213} \boxed{54\ 213} + \bigodot{100} \bigodot{100} \bigodot{100} \bigodot{100}$$

High School

The summer Patricia was 10, we vacationed in Pennsylvania. One day, we took a detour from learning how to make pretzels at an Amish bakery and went to Hershey Park. It's a theme park where all the rides are made out of chocolate. Patricia and I weren't fans of the big roller coasters, but we did get great satisfaction from going on the middle-sized, kiddie versions of them. Never loops. But steel coasters were OK.

This place presented a real dilemma. For the first time ever, we were faced with a kid-sized version of a looping steel roller coaster. Being the good dad, I encouraged Patricia to go on it with me. She reluctantly agreed. As we left the starting gate, things were looking good. Up the long clicking ramp. Still pretty good. Down the first incline. Big smile. Going into the first loop, Patricia shouted, "Dad, make it stop!" I told her calmly that I was unable to do that. Going into the next curve, Patricia shouted even louder, "Dad, you can do anything. Make it stop!" It made me feel good that Patricia had this much confidence in my abilities. Unfortunately, I wasn't able to deliver. That day. Or again. When she really needed it.

∞

Those first two days of ninth grade were a disaster. The weekend was worse. It took another 24 hours to get Patricia back into the hospital. Things were so desperate on Sunday night that I called the emergency pager number at Raymond Counseling.

No one called me back.

On Monday morning, I was able to get in touch with the office staff and make an emergency appointment with our nurse practitioner, Carol, for later that day. When we met, she expressed real concern for Patricia's situation. She said to double Patricia's Prozac, providing, of course, we made it home.

Next, we were off to a therapy appointment with Deb. I sat down to read the tabloids while Patricia went in to see her. (Remember, I didn't choose this place.) Within a couple of minutes, Deb dragged me into the back. "Patricia is not safe." "She needs to go to EMH." "Why did Carol let you out of her office?" "Did you even talk to her about how Patricia was feeling?" *I think so. And we're here. So she can talk with you. Her therapist.*

I learned something new that day: Even if you have access to a licensed nurse practitioner (sort of like a psychiatrist—except without all those years of medical school), and a licensed clinical social worker (one flavor of psychotherapist), when your kid is melting down, they can't actually help. *Ugh.*

We went back to EMH—emergency mental health. Deb called them to say we were on our way. Didn't help. Even going to the right hospital didn't change anything. We just ended up at the end of a long line of people who needed "an evaluation."

But something was new. Because this was the right hospital, they had a special section with a special milieu for our particular kind of clientele: Locked cabinets. Locked doors. Mesh in the windows.

If this is intended to give a sense of comfort and security, the hospitals need to rethink their intent. The first thing that happens is all your stuff: cell phone, keys, wallet, briefcase, pen, fingernail clippers, and every other appendage to daily living, gets locked up in a file cabinet. For those of us who can't think ourselves out of a paper bag without a pencil and pad of paper to doodle on, this leaves us incredibly vulnerable. The second thing is you find yourself locked in a room with one or two other families—usually one that includes a teenage girl dressed all in black, with piercings in places you never thought needed piercing—watching those shows on Nick at Nite you would never in a million years let your child watch—EVEN WHEN SHE WAS 14.

Grandmothers. There were grandmothers, too. Panicked ones. Grandmothers who clearly didn't want to be watching these shows either—not the ones on TV, and certainly not the one going on around them. They sat there, trying to be invisible, all the while their eyes darting back to their charge.

This went on for hours. And hours.

When it was finally time for the evaluation, I wasn't really prepared to advocate for my child. Patricia had neglected to tell me we might be going to EMH when we left the house earlier in the day, so all my important papers were still at home. Even details like medication doses. Not sure. Those answers were locked up in my notebook in the file cabinet. And I didn't have anything to write on, or with, so I couldn't write anything down or doodle my questions into cohesive thoughts. All for the want of my locked-up pen.

Ultimately, it was decided that Patricia would go back to Patriot Medical. They would help sort out her medications. An ambulance was called and we set off for Wellesley at 3:30 a.m. I parked in the lot and made my way to the Children's Psychiatric Unit to meet Patricia. I knew the way. It took a while for her to show up at the nurse's station. When she finally made it, she told me that they had diverted her to the Emergency Room in order to get a medical screening from the new hospital before they would let her onto the unit. Patricia said that the doctor who administered it told her she could solve all her problems if she just found religion. That she didn't really need to be here. Patricia went off to bed in the quiet room just as the sun started up. I seethed all the way home. And, later in the day, I seethed all the way back.

We met with Dr. Chase again. He told us that the social worker was still out on maternity leave, so we were stuck with him again. I expressed my displeasure with the religion comment from his doctor.

This hospital stay was very different. Patricia already knew all the words to the songs. So did I. Patricia's goal was to have the hospital adjust her medicines so she would feel better—instead of worse. The hospital's goal was to stabilize her and send her home in four days. If you've been paying attention, there is a conflict here. The outpatient people, Carol and Deb, sent us to the hospital to get the meds fixed. The hospital was prepared to stabilize her and send her back into the caring arms of the outpatient people—

the same ones who sent us to the hospital in the first place. Something's wrong. Big time.

And the problem is bigger than just my kid.

Patricia spent another 10 days in the hospital.

The hospital psychiatrist agreed with Carol about increasing the Prozac. I made a fresh copy of a blank side-effect checklist. The staff went off to deal with new cases and left Patricia to fend for herself. Patricia was the ideal patient. The staff loved her. They asked. She did. But if they didn't ask, sometime in the last month (or year), she'd lost her ability to do for herself. They were too busy to notice. Patricia was too shut-down to say anything.

We sat at the end of her bed and talked. Quiet thoughts. Just like we had for all those years. School. This week's viola lesson. What friends might say. But I could see changes brewing. We started checking things off the side-effect list again. Rapidly. And this time, the event that precipitated getting the checkmark was much more disturbing than the last time. She was having trouble sitting still. We'd be talking, and, all of a sudden, she'd stand up, tip her head to the ceiling, smile, start hopping up and down, spinning slowly in a circle, talking a mile a minute. I liked the smiling part, but I'd never seen any of those other things in my child before. I informed the nursing staff.

Despite the smiles, Patricia became more and more unhappy. She was frustrated with the hospital. There wasn't anything new. She tried to work on her safety plan, but everyone loved it. "Best one I've ever seen." Dr. Chase, who by this time had been doing two jobs for a month longer than he'd been doing them last time, wasn't participating in groups the way he did the last time she was there. Patricia, who had had a month to think about what was going on inside her, and who was just beginning to identify some real issues that needed airing—or venting—was aware that the group experience she was getting from the recreational therapist aide was different than the one she could be getting from the Doctor of Psychology who was busy covering for a social worker out on maternity leave. This bothered Patricia. She was trying to get better. Why wouldn't they help her?

Patricia reported having dreams. Remembered, for the first time. Vivid dreams. Some disturbing. Others comforting. One about Zorkans attacking earth: Patricia borrowed a spaceship from

NASA and successfully fought them off. I got to help. And then we donated a captured Zorkan ship to NASA. She dreamt she could sing. In tune. And there was one dream where she was sitting in a tree. Brian Sculthorpe came down from above and sat next to her. He gave her a hug and said, "It will be OK. You can get through it." I informed the nursing staff.

Patricia started hearing voices. Voices? She talked with a nurse about this. No, she didn't know what they were saying.

On day three, sitting at the end of her bed, Patricia next to me, she got anxious and squirmy again. She hit me. For the first time in her entire life. She hit me. Just an elbow to the ribs. But hard. It hurt. She was already teary. Her expression didn't change. I chose not to react, but again, I informed the nursing staff.

The next day, Patricia was worse. Decompensating. Something that wasn't supposed to happen in the hospital. She should be getting better. Getting stable. So she could come home. As we sat at the end of her bed, Patricia asked me quietly if I would help her break a window. To get her out of there. And smuggle her home. So she could kill herself.

This got the nurse's attention. And the psychiatrist's.

It got my attention, too. This is another one of those things a father doesn't want to hear from his perfect child. She was serious. There wasn't any smirk. No sense about how this would be another one of our great adventures. Just sadness. And terror. She had a problem. She knew that I knew how to solve them. She asked for my help. But it wasn't a cry for help. It was real. She wasn't talking to the father who loved her. And at that moment, she wasn't the perfect child, either. Just someone who needed to get from point A to point B, but didn't know the path to get her there. But did know she was sitting next to the one guy in the world who she believed had the power to stop a speeding roller coaster. Mid-loop.

There is a difference between wanting to die and wanting to be dead. Patricia wanted to be dead. That would have made her happy. She might not have been too thrilled about what it would take to get there, but it was very clear she wanted to be dead. Relief. Relief from something awful inside her. Something more terrible than what could be overcome by logic, or love, or family, or by a seemingly happy life.

I had been comforted, for a while, believing Patricia was safe. Because she knew what suicide did to a family and a town. That comfort was shattered when she took those 40 Motrin pills the night of her first hospitalization. But there were still some shards of hope left. Until now. Now I was beginning to understand. It wasn't about how her death would affect anyone. Not her family. Not her town. Not even herself. She didn't care how her death would affect her family. Because she wasn't thinking about us. She didn't care how her death would affect her town or her friends. Because she wasn't thinking about them, either. She didn't even care how her death would affect her. She'd be dead. But she didn't care. She didn't care about being dead. What she cared about was being alive. The problem was being alive. Not being dead. She was so overwhelmed with sadness, she just wanted out. It's not all about me. It's all about me not wanting to be me anymore.

This is what I think committing to suicide is all about.

That day, I saw the dark for the first time. But I still didn't know what I was looking at. And I still didn't know what we'd done to cause it.

∞

Brian Sculthorpe "committed suicide." Those are the words people use. Other, more knowledgeable people might use the phrase, "completed suicide." This is used to differentiate between an "attempted suicide" and the real thing. The circumstances leading up to Brian's death can never be known, because he was the only one there. He did something. He ended up dead. Maybe his intent was to be dead. Or maybe it was something else. To scare himself. To scare others. Or an accident. For him, it doesn't matter. For the rest of us, it probably shouldn't matter either.

We were starting to learn more about Patricia's suicide attempts. We already knew she wasn't expecting to wake up that Tuesday after she "took 14 pain pills." We knew she was trying to kill herself during the few seconds when she "took 40 Motrin pills." Patricia was beginning to admit that there was another incident, with some more pills, somewhere between the 14 and 40.

Originally, we thought Kate's stroke was the traumatic event that led Patricia to take those pills. It may have been, but it doesn't really matter, either. Because we learned Patricia had been thinking about this even before then. If not that, it would have been something else. Maybe bad fathering. We learned later, that on the evening before the stroke, Patricia was "contemplating suicide." The next morning, when the sirens permeated our quiet street, Patricia thought they were coming for her. She thought she had "committed to suicide" the night before, and they were coming to pick up the pieces that next morning. Maybe she thought she was dead. Or maybe she thought she was alive. In either case, her preference would have been the former.

"Commit to suicide" is the term I think matters the most. Brian "completed suicide." We'll never know if he "committed to suicide." Patricia did. At least twice. The first two times she took some pills, went to bed, and didn't expect to wake up. Ever. And I was beginning to get to know a child who was working very hard to stay alive, but who also believed her quickest relief would be realized by "committing to suicide" again.

This is not the happy place a father wants to be.

Patricia's importance at the hospital changed. She moved out of the chorus and back to a lead. The psychiatrist spent more time with her. This was interfering with Dr. Chase's plans to stabilize her and send her home. The depressed child they had diagnosed a month ago was now exhibiting signs of "mania." Mania. Another word I didn't know. More research. But Patricia had already done the research. Bipolar. The new word for Manic Depressive Disorder. When the mood swings from depression to mania, you get bipolar. Patricia had already diagnosed herself with that.

Patricia's diagnosis changed today. It now is:
Bipolar Disorder, NOS
Anxiety Disorder, NOS.

And when the diagnosis changes, you get to change the medicines, too. We added Lithium and Seroquel, both powerful drugs. They have a whole slew of new side-effects. Weight gain. Headaches. Increased paranoia. Or you can develop tardive dyskinesia, an incurable disease that shows up out of nowhere and manifests itself as involuntary, repetitive movements. You twitch.

It wasn't out yet, but Heath Ledger skillfully demonstrated this phenomenon with his tongue protrusions when he played the Joker in the new Batman movie, *The Dark Knight*. Right before he succumbed to too many prescription drugs.

So we took it slowly. Patricia's medicines bumped up another couple of times.

The result was remarkable. Patricia's mood turned right around. She felt better. We started talking about going home. And not because her four days were up, but because she was actually better. We talked about this with Dr. Chase. He told us that most bipolar children spend eight years trying to figure out what is going on before they get their bipolar diagnosis. Our child managed to do it in eight weeks. *Go, Patricia.*

During the few days it took to get her medicine "up to a therapeutic level," a new but relatively self-explanatory phrase, we revisited some topics with Dr. Chase and the psychiatrist. These new dreams interested them. We talked about Patricia when she was in grade school and the fantastic stories she told. Just characters. They'd play out stories in her head. "Do you hear voices?" *No.* "Do you see things other people don't see?" *No.* "Is anyone telling you to do something?" *No.* "Have you been feeling anxious or panicky?" *Yes.* "Do you think people are watching you?" *Yes.* "Do you think others can control your thoughts?" *Probably not.* "Do you think you can control other's thoughts?" *Maybe.*

Probably just the new meds.

If I'd been paying attention a little better, I would have wondered about the answer to that first question. The one about the voices. Hadn't Patricia reported hearing voices just a few days before? But she didn't know what they were saying? Maybe I missed it. Or maybe I was focusing too much on her reports of feeling better.

∞

When the hope of discharge began to glimmer at the end of the tunnel, it was time to schedule some appointments with Carol and Deb. Because Patricia's medications were becoming more ominous, many of the people we were starting to meet spoke strongly about the need to have a real child psychiatrist. Carol Sherman was a nurse practitioner. Not a psychiatrist. I still didn't know the difference. But I did know that I'd choose a competent nurse practitioner over an unsatisfactory psychiatrist any day. We'd already had one of those. Still, the advice was to find a real child psychiatrist.

Because Dr. Chase was still doing two jobs, it was up to me to make the after-discharge appointments. Instead of trying the proven unreturned-phone-call-technique, I decided to drive down to Raymond Counseling and talk with the receptionist. I explained that Patricia was in the hospital, she was a patient of Carol Sherman, she needed an appointment with her in order to be discharged from the hospital, but even though we really, really liked Carol (because she was the only one who ever actually talked to Patricia), we were being counseled to find her a real child psychiatrist, and do you have any of those here we could make an appointment with, so she can come home, please? The receptionist listened to my story. She said there was only one child psychiatrist at the clinic. He was the director. He wasn't accepting new patients. But she'd see if they had any ideas. She promised to call me back.

She did.

Dr. Goodman, the director of the clinic, agreed to see Patricia until she was stable. When the time was right, we could transfer back to Carol. We made an appointment. He's still her doctor. We're still working on prolonged stability.

On the morning of her tenth day in the hospital, my cell phone rang. It was Dr. Chase calling to say that Patricia was ready to come home. He wanted me to come get her. *When?* Now.

This presented a dilemma. A big one. Because I was busy. Remember the tree? From the storm during the last hospital stay? Well, I was standing in a field, one town away from home, watching that hundred-year-old oak get turned into lumber. I had found a guy with a portable sawmill big enough to cut it up. He had just finished the first cut. The prospect of shutting this whole operation down was overwhelming. Normally, I'd say yes to a doctor, but I couldn't today. Because I was busy.

During Patricia's previous hospitalization, I learned something I was able to use to resolve this situation. I knew that Patricia wasn't going anywhere until and unless I showed up to pick her up. I told Dr. Chase I was busy. Simple as that. That I would be there when I could. It made me feel like a criminal.

I spent a pleasant couple of hours watching the tree get chopped up into what would ultimately become our new dining room table. After stashing the boards at home in the garage, I went to get Patricia.

∞

After a second psychiatric hospitalization, you start to win things: Prizes. Like a game show. Everything is free, but you still have to show up and play in order to take home each prize. The first one was a referral to CAP, the now-defunct Massachusetts Collaborative Assessment Program. These people saved Patricia's life. Without it, we never would have figured out how to access any of the services that kept her safe while we tried to figure out what to do.

Here's how it worked: A woman (who reminded me of Mary Poppins) showed up at our home. She had a clipboard. She started taking names. She interviewed the children, Patricia and Beth. She interviewed Kate and me. I think she looked around for dust on the mantle. And probably checked out what was left in the medicine cabinet after The Purging. We signed release forms giving her permission to talk to all of Patricia's new providers. She peeked at our tax return.

A few days later, she brought a "friend" with her to visit. This was a mom whose only qualification was that she had a kid who had gone through her own version of what Patricia was struggling with. She was carefully chosen. A happy ending—or at least a palatable one—was guaranteed. Here we were talking to a mother who had been through something horrible. Something like we were just beginning to go through. And her kid wasn't dead. She talked about how hard it was for her. That she didn't know anything or where to turn. She persevered. We could too. She could help. "Call me if you have any questions. Here's my card." *I don't know what to ask.* "You will."

She left us with a list of parent support groups in our area. There was one in Worcester and another in Gardner. I went to both. I tried to sit quietly in the corner. To watch. But they made me talk. Most importantly, they made me feel as if it was OK to talk. Like I wasn't the only one who ever found themselves in an impossible situation with absolutely no idea of what to do. I still go. Nearly everything I've learned on this adventure, I learned at a parent support meeting.

∞

Everyone who goes through a CAP assessment also wins a neatly bound report to take home. Ours is 32 pages long. A brick. It describes the kid, the situation, the players. All in extremely frank and clinical language. To paraphrase it, it says we're screwed. Big time. Patricia is struggling. And we should expect some difficult times ahead, particularly relating to school. Because Patricia presents so well and has historically excelled in school, we might have trouble convincing her teachers she really is sick and entitled to some accommodations. It turns out this is a double-edged sword. In order for any accommodation to work, both the school and the child need to agree that it is necessary. And reasonable. Who knew Patricia might be the bigger problem?

In talking with Brenda Harris, Patricia's guidance counselor, it became clear Patricia was not welcome back at school until there was a Meeting. They wanted to make sure that Patricia would be safe at school and that the school would be safe from Patricia. I had already signed release forms, so they were allowed to talk with each other. They did. The day after Patricia was discharged from the hospital, there was a 504 Meeting at the school. 504 is a section of the Americans with Disabilities Act. It says that no one with a disability can be excluded from participating in federally funded programs or activities. Apparently, school is one of those things. The 504 process sets forth accommodations designed to allow Patricia to participate fully, despite her disability. A 504 Plan is different from and less comprehensive than an Individual Education Plan, or IEP. We didn't get one of those until later.

Patricia was at this meeting. So were Kate and I. The other side of the table was loaded: the school's 504 coordinator, the nurse, the school psychologist, and the assistant principal. Brenda Harris sat between us, as if she were the referee. We were new at this, but we did know we had the right to bring others to the table with us. We could hire an advocate. We could hire a lawyer. We could bring a friend. Or my sister. We decided to go it alone and see what happened. And to let Patricia's illness speak for itself.

It did.

There are two parts to a 504 Plan. The first one asks if there is a handicap which affects a major life activity. There was. Yes. Definitely. No question. *Drat.* The next part describes the reasonable accommodations to address this disability:

Patricia's 504 Accommodations

- ☐ *Allow student access to guidance counselor, school psychologist, administrators, or school nurse when needed.*
- ☐ *Allow snacks and drinks in class for medical reasons.*
- ☐ *Abbreviated day/excused tardy for doctor appointments.*
- ☐ *Allow extended time as needed for homework, written assignments, and long term projects.*
- ☐ *Provide supplemental teacher notes when absent and allow use of a study-buddy for notes and/or homework.*

We also made modifications to Patricia's schedule.

Back in the spring, before anyone except Patricia knew anything was up, the "high school transition system," with all its momentum and cogs, put Patricia into six honors classes. You know, the ones for the smart kids. I was a little surprised, her being only in the 88th percentile and all, but I was very proud of her. I was also scared. During his infamous Coffee and Chats, Dennis, the middle school principal, had warned us that if this happened, the good parent would think very carefully before approving such a plan. Children need to have lives in addition to school. Dennis was adamant. I believed him. So we took her out of honors Latin, honors Algebra II and honors science.

This change already had one consequence we didn't comprehend yet. It had to do with Algebra II. In fifth grade, Patricia took a test that placed her on the fast-track for math in middle school. She zoomed right through it, doing very well, just as we expected. However, when it came time for high school, she was already finished with freshman math. Therefore, being in honors Algebra II put her into a class of sophomores who liked math. The real problem happened when Patricia moved down a notch to regular college-prep Algebra II. Now instead of being in a class of sophomores who liked math, she was in a class of juniors who hated math. Even though she was a freshman, Patricia was by far the smartest kid in the class. Even with her disability.

As a result of the 504 Meeting, honors history was downgraded to college-prep history. Honors strings was dropped. This would give Patricia time to catch up. We were pleased.

∞

The next thing the CAP Assessment won for Patricia was a referral to the Massachusetts Department of Mental Health, DMH. In Massachusetts, children only get "picked up," meaning receive services, by either DMH or the Department of Children & Families, DCF (formerly known as the Department of Social Services). Never both. If you apply to one, they might say you don't qualify. If you press them and can demonstrate a need, their second line of defense might be to say that the other agency is more qualified to provide services. Go talk to them. The result is that the child can get the run-around for quite some time before anyone feels the least bit obligated to actually do anything. The beauty of the CAP program was it short-circuits everything. Not only does it determine whether there is a need, but it also decides which agency will provide the services. And it's voluntary for the family, but not for the State. If you agree with the recommendation, the agency must take you on as a client.

Deciding what to do after winning this referral is one of those monumental decisions you'd rather not be faced with. If we say no, then the child still isn't sick. If we say yes, then she will be forever labeled as a client of the Department of Mental Health. Stigmatized. No turning back. Which would you choose? Sick? Or fine? The problem was that Patricia wasn't fine. We chose DMH.

Hooking up with DMH gave us "peoples."

We were starting to form a team. A Treatment Team. We were on it: Mom and Dad. Patricia was on it too. And we were very lucky for that. I sensed at the time, and later experiences confirmed, when the kid isn't invested in getting better, the kid doesn't. Brenda Harris was on the team. So were Deb and Dr. Goodman. But they weren't real members yet. They were important, but because they were isolated and shielded by receptionists and scheduled appointments, they weren't able to participate and be as reactive as we needed. They had very specific roles, and during appointments with them, time was spent doing their thing, but they were not available to help ruminate over the big picture and make strategic plans. And things were starting to move faster. Decisions needed to be made. We couldn't wait for a week for the next appointment to sneak in a question at the end of a session. And even if we could, we wouldn't know what to ask.

For a while, we were under the impression that the staff at the hospital, the psychiatrist, and the combination psychologist/social worker, were on our Team. They were the ones who knew what was going on and what needed doing. It turns out that once the discharge papers are signed by the "responsible" parent, services stop. They go on with the business of treating their patients who are still in the hospital. Their only obligation is to write a report. When it's done, in a few months, and with the right forms, you can get a copy of it too. But it is never available in a timely fashion when it could actually do any good.

All of a sudden, we had peoples: a DMH case manager, a DMH flexible services coordinator, and a youth support worker. People to call and ask questions. People who wanted to meet and help us figure out what to do. What to do first. And then what to do next.

$\begin{array}{cc}54\\107\end{array}$ $\begin{array}{cc}54\\107\end{array}$ 200   200   100

$$-\ \text{100} + \text{100} + \text{54}_{107} + \text{25} + \text{54}_{107} + \text{25} + \text{100} + \text{25}\ \text{25}$$

$$+\ \text{25} + \text{25} - \text{50} + \text{100} + \text{100} + \text{1} - \text{1} + \text{0} + \text{100}$$

Changes

Freshman year was a time of changes. We were settling into a new routine, filled (we thought) with lots of activities to keep Patricia busy: Viola lessons. Destination Imagination. Deb. And regular visits to Dr. Goodman. We had our own looping-roller-coaster ride of medication changes over the next several months. Nothing worked. And every time we changed something, if one thing got better, we ended up with two new problems.

To demonstrate this, we are going to go through this time twice. First we'll look at it from a medication point of view. Then we'll go back and talk about the kid. They really are two different stories. Patricia began this time taking five pills—the ones shown at the end of the last chapter. During this chapter, she will have eleven medication changes—adding fifteen pills and eliminating three. You can play along by watching the graphics at the beginning of the chapter. When we are all done, she will be taking ten pills, the ones shown at the end. Just for a while, we'll do some math with the meds and watch them change along the way.

∞

Seroquel is a wonderful drug. Not only was Patricia getting *to* sleep, she was also sleeping through the night—which means I could move from my place on the floor next to her bed and back to my own room. Patricia awoke rested. Refreshed. But clumsy. She would walk into things. Fall up the stairs. She was getting bruises on her bruises. We complained to Dr. Goodman. He eliminated the morning Seroquel.

Stop morning Seroquel, because of clumsiness.   —   (100)

= (54/107) (54/107) (200) (200)

That solved the clumsiness problem. But a new one came up. The Seroquel had been doing something else, too. Maybe something beneficial. Because when it went away, Patricia started making comments like, "My mind hasn't shut up since I stopped taking the morning Seroquel." And, "My ears are crowded." *What does that mean?* She didn't know. She was having more vivid dreams, "Dreams of secret experiments and shape-shifting crows watching everything." This stuff was all new to me. I'd never heard anything like this before.

We talked more about the fantastic stories Patricia used to tell us when she was in elementary school. She described them as "characters" who talked among themselves. Sort of like a play. They'd talk. She'd listen. Lots of drama. Maybe like a soap opera on TV, or *Beverly Hills, 90210* (even though we never watched either). My sense from Patricia was that it was an ongoing story. Today we had Episode One. Tomorrow was Episode Two. Patricia said the stories were interesting, but repetitive. *Repetitive? What does that mean? Maybe I should ask.*

Being the good dad, I helped Patricia pass this on to Deb. After their session, Deb added some clinical language: "Repetitive auditory hallucinations with homicidal themes." I hadn't heard that part. *Uh-oh.*

I passed this along to Dr. Goodman.

Add more evening Seroquel, for mood and sleep.   +   (100)

= (54/107) (54/107) (200) (200) (100)

The side-effects started to get interesting. Hands and feet were tingly. Ears ringing—when going from a loud place to a quiet place—or when moving from one place to another where there is a change in temperature. Dizzy. Off balance. Black spots. She started to see in black and white shapes. Little twitches. Then bigger twitches. Woke up—couldn't see. Drink more water—but wasn't she already drinking plenty of water yesterday? Sight returns.

Headaches. Brutal headaches. Twitching leg. Dreams are gone. Trouble getting to sleep at night. Brutally tired during the day. She needed help standing up. And when she did, she said, "My stomach just disappeared." Carbohydrate cravings. Donuts. Smiles. But sad, too. Sad while smiling. And jumping around. Mania?

Add more Lithium, for mania. + (54/107)

Start Lamictal, to stabilize mood. + (25)

= (54/107) (54/107) (54/107) (200) (200) (100) (25)

Now we had to watch out for a rash. If you get the rash, stop the Lamictal. If not, it will kill you. Weren't we trying to prevent that? And stop eating grapefruit. Who actually eats grapefruit, anyway? *Patricia.* Who actually missed not being able to eat grapefruit? *Patricia.*

More technical terms from Deb. "Passive suicidal ideations." *What does that mean?* No plan. But thinking about it. *Don't you come up with a plan by thinking about it?*

The characters quietly disappeared. Then, "Like a bucket of water, they came back."

Add more Lithium, for mania. + (54/107)

Add more Lamictal, to stabilize mood. + (25)

Add more Seroquel, for mood and sleep. + (100)

= (54/107) (54/107) (54/107) (54/107) (300) (300) (25) (25)

Weight gain became an issue. Patricia had always been a little underweight, but at her annual physical, she just crossed the fiftieth percentile on the growth and development chart. She wasn't overweight, yet, but she had gained 40 pounds in four months. Clothes didn't fit anymore. And Patricia was reluctant to admit she needed larger ones.

Even though the characters aren't there so often, when they are, they are harder to ignore. More headaches. Every day. Motrin helps—for a while.

Add more Lamictal, to stabilize mood.   +   (25) (25)

Start Topamax, for mood and to reduce appetite.   +   (25)

= (54/107) (54/107) (54/107) (54/107) (300) (300) (100) (25)

And stop taking Motrin—it increases the effect of the Lithium. I wondered why you wouldn't start taking Motrin and reduce the Lithium if you could get the same effect. No one could answer my question.

And watch out for kidney stones or eye problems. Blacking out and blurry vision is OK, just other kinds of eye problems. Good, because we still had blackouts and blurry vision.

Tired. Couldn't concentrate. Couldn't remember what she was doing. Couldn't find a place in the house to get away from the noise.

Left pinky toe tingling. Felt like it was going to fall off. Then the bridge of her nose and both ears started tingling. She said it felt like she was wearing glasses.

More concentration problems. Trouble with a history quiz. Class was too loud.

"My head feels tired, but my brain doesn't, but I know it will soon."

Tingling knee, down into the shin.

It was nearly winter. Trouble with the cold. Is there a difference between a shiver and a twitch? Not sure.

Add more Topamax, for mood.   +   (25)

= (54/107) (54/107) (54/107) (54/107) (300) (300) (100) (50)

Shooting muscle pain in both arms. All day. Headache. Water doesn't help.

"My soul hurts."

Thoughts. Mean. Mad at everything. Suicidal ideations. Urge to cut. "I know this is wrong. I'm 97% sure I am stronger than this."

More dog walks. Particularly when Patricia is upset. But that's a coping skill, so it's OK, right?

Tears. "A flood of emotions." "All good."

Now we had to deal with the idea that tears aren't always bad. Burning eyes. That's different from blurry.

Stop Topamax, for mood.   — (50)

= (54/107) (54/107) (54/107) (54/107) (300) (300) (100)

Better. Until Deb told us not to leave her alone for a while. Very concerned. No unsupervised dog walks.

Tears.

Dr. Goodman told us to renegotiate the no-dog-walking policy with Deb. Called her. Left a message. No response. Called again. No response. Next week. OK with Deb.

Still tingly.

Almost blacked-out getting out of bed in the morning.

More suicidal ideations.

I noticed Patricia would count sprinkler heads, ceiling lights, and floor tiles. Was this important? Who needed to know? And whose job was it to tell them? Mine? Patricia's?

Characters are still present. But just a little. "They don't bug me. And I can tune them out."

Start morning Lamictal, to stabilize mood.   + (100)

= (54/107) (54/107) (54/107) (54/107) (300) (300) (7248)

Shaking. One day at lunch, a classmate Patricia had never met, commented to her that she was shaking. So much for blending in. Ears ringing, but not too disruptive. Inside of forearm hurts. Left foot trouble. Comfortable when twisted in, but uncomfortable when in normal alignment.

More characters. "But I can ignore them when I'm talking to people."

Headaches. More shaking. Water helps.

Unable to swallow. "I thought I was going to choke." Better.

Sobbing in bed.

Characters gone.

Lost words.

Twitching.

Easily frustrated.

Urge to cut.

Tingling. Arms, legs, and torso, "Like big raindrops hitting your skin before you get wet."

Panicked. Jittery. Hopping from foot to foot. More tears.

Trouble breathing in gym. Maybe it's just asthma. She's had that.

"I feel dark. Inside my soul."

Add more Lamictal, to stabilize mood.   + (100)

Start Abilify, for depression.   + (1)

= (54/107) (54/107) (54/107) (54/107) (300) (300) (150) (150) (1)

Ears ringing. Loud.

Shaking. Lots of shaking.

Spots. Dizzy. Reports of waking up in the night.

Characters are including Patricia in their conversations. Not command, but pointed comments directed at Patricia.

Stuffy ears. Blotchy vision.

Patricia reports that, "The new medicine is making me feel different." "Like sandbags on my head and arms and everywhere." "Everything is dark." "It's like being under a glacier, only not as flat." "Like I'm full of water." "Like everything is not as bright." "Like I'm wearing sunglasses."

Dr. Goodman didn't like any of this. Neither did we.

Stop Abilify, for depression.   — (1)

Start Ativan, PRN, for anxiety.   + (0)

= (54/107) (54/107) (54/107) (54/107) (300) (300) (150) (150) (0)

"PRN" is a new term. It means to take it when you need it. You know, when things aren't going well. *Does that mean she takes it all the time?* Wait. It's only for anxiety. *So maybe she only needs to take it when she's awake?* We had a lot of anxiety.

"I feel safe, but I don't want to be alive."

Add more Seroquel, for mood and sleep.   + (100)

= (54/107) (54/107) (54/107) (54/107) (300) (300) (100) (150) (150) (0)

That's enough medication details. They are getting in the way of our story.

∞

If you haven't guessed, we're heading back to the hospital. It will take another week or so to get there, but we're on the way. Things get worse. If you can believe it. But before we make it there, we are going to rewind to the beginning of freshman year and watch things play out from a life-perspective rather than just focusing on the meds and their side-effects. Changes in how you manage life is a side-effect too. Is it from the disease? Or is it from the medicine? Remember that Patricia had been a kid before. She knew how to do things. How to make friends. How to play the viola. How to be a sister. A member of a family. A member of a team. And how to be a person who excelled at almost everything she put her mind to.

We began to lose these things. The things that let Patricia be normal were starting to disappear. "Shut-down" was a new phrase that fit any one of a number of different circumstances. It described what happened when Patricia no longer knew how to react when exposed to all the everyday parts of life she used to handle so well.

In the couple of days between the time we came back from our cruise and the start of freshman year, the anxiety level started to rise. Patricia got a form letter from the new principal. His letter made it clear that he had some ideas on how to run a high school and he was prepared to implement new rules starting on day one.

The school was undergoing a renovation and expansion project that dwarfed any of my home remodeling undertakings. It was almost done, but just like me, they had been saying that for years. During this particular phase, many of the already-too-small corridors would be barricaded. Getting from class to class might be a challenge, but because of strict state mandates regarding time on learning, the interval between classes would be reduced, instead of extended. "I expect you to be to class on time." Also, snacks, gum, and drinks in the classroom have gotten a little out of control, so those will no longer be permitted.

Because of the Lithium, Patricia needed to drink lots of water. It wasn't clear whether water was allowed in the classroom, and if so, could you actually take a sip in class or did you need to wait until you were out in the hallways between classes? We asked two different people. And got two different answers. Neither came from someone Patricia was willing to bet a detention on.

Our visit to Brenda Harris, the guidance counselor, on the day before school started went a long way to mitigate Patricia's anxiety. She made it through the first day of school. Barely. There was nowhere near enough time to get to some of her classes on time. Some hallways were clogged with so many students that no one moved anywhere. Others had fewer pedestrians, but the current was going the wrong way. Those were worse. Patricia decided not to drink anything those first days. The water policy was being interpreted differently by each teacher. But after the first day of school, it didn't matter. With that new sleeping pill with the metallic-taste side-effect, drinking anything was not an option. After that, she landed in the hospital again.

∞

Patricia's first hospitalization happened during school vacation. It didn't affect her social life very much. She wasn't ever missing. There were a couple of calls from friends, but they were satisfied with the response that Patricia was out of town for a few days. After some careful thought, Patricia decided to tell her best friend where she was and how she ended up there. It went surprisingly well. I called the friend's mom first, told her Patricia was in the hospital, and explained the situation. I said that with her permission, Patricia would like to call her daughter and share what was going on. I asked the mom for one consideration: That she call me and give me a heads-up if she ever found out that her daughter decided she could no longer be Patricia's friend. The mom was very understanding. She promised to let me know if the time ever came. Patricia called her friend. She was understanding, too. Their friendship survived. This was a major milestone.

Missing school for the second hospitalization was more troublesome. She was missed. Lots more friends and acquaintances noticed she was absent during days 4 through 14 of the new school year. Patricia lamented about this in the hospital. What would she say? What would her friends say? What would her real friends say? And what would the others say? The hospital staff didn't have any worthy ideas. This was not acceptable.

Finally, Patricia and I came up with an idea. I talked with Dr. Chase about it. He thought it was OK. Next we needed to ask Kate, mom, if it was all right with her. She agreed. The plan was that if asked, Patricia would say she was stressed out and landed in the hospital. This is a true statement. If pressed, she would say she was stressed out because her mom had a stroke. "How would you handle it if your mom had a stroke?" This statement was designed to end the discussion. It worked. Just once. Because it was only needed once. Patricia's "real friends" only needed the first version. The "fake friend" needed the second one. Patricia felt very good at how easy her friends made it for her. And she wasn't surprised at which "friend" needed the long version.

∞

"Freaking out" is another term we need to add along with "shut-down." Because being shut-down goes along with, or leads to, freaking out. Unless, of course, you are too shut-down to freak out. Crowds were becoming an issue. One friend was OK, but too many people—friends, family, or strangers in the same room—became overwhelming. Parties, which used to be fun, were a veritable Petri dish for anxiety. Knowing what to do about it was no longer obvious.

You're at a party at a friend's house. Things are getting a little too much. What do you do? Go to the bathroom? Before you know it, someone needs to use it. Go into the other room? What if it's "off limits?" What will they say when they find you there? Go outside? Then what? Walk home? Talk to the friend who is hosting the party? What do you say? Talk to the host's mom? What do you say then? Call dad? *I hope so.* Before the parties stopped, luckily, Patricia usually chose talking to the mom. Maybe a call to dad to come pick her up. Or maybe just a Benadryl to help calm down. Thankfully, the moms always vetoed the walk-yourself-home idea. No matter what Patricia chose, it always started with debilitating anxiety. But to resolve it, it always required an action more threatening than just shutting-down and sticking it out. I went and picked her up lots of times that year. When I saw the look on her face when I got there, terror being replaced by relief, I wondered what could be going on that was so awful she needed to pull whatever strings she had to pull in order to get out of there rather than just wait it out. More than anything, I was proud of her.

Times with family and family friends were just as unpredictable. Knowing what to do and how to react was a big dilemma. We were at a cookout one day at a public park. Patricia had had enough. She asked if she could walk home. I said no—we were 50 miles from home. What if she hadn't asked? And what were we supposed to do then? Leave early? What would we say? What would the people with us think? We parents were in the same predicament as the kid. Eventually, when Kate was able to drive again, we brought two cars. It just made it easier.

When we were closer to home, what to do presented a similar quandary. We were at friends. She'd had enough. She asked if she could walk home. This time, I said yes. When we came home, she was teary and mopey. She sat by my chair. By now, that made me nervous. The next day she handed me another poem:

> On a cold night in winter
> A girl steps out of her house
> She walks down the road
> She last snuck out two months ago
> But a lot has changed.
> Yes, the cold harsh wind still blows
> but this time the wind doesn't carry sand
> This time it carries snow
> Little ice chips
> Digging into her skin
> like a frozen shovel
> The wind, whipping around
> Picks up her dark locks
> And throws them to the side
> exposing her ear.
> Her light sweatshirt
> Barely creates a barrier
> against the elements
> So while she walks
> by the Honey Farms

She stops inside
And begs the man
behind the counter
to let her stay
but he doesn't yield
and he throws her outside
So she walks down the road
and stops at the beach
and curls up in a ball
Lying down
She slowly forgets
why she has to stay awake
She is standing
in a dark tunnel
with a light at the end
something's telling her
that the place with the light
is warm and safe
a good place to walk to
a good place to be
The police find her
just as dawn breaks
but they can't find a pulse
they cry for her
they cry for her family
and what they will have to go through
And when the family comes
To file the missing report
and they hear the awful news
they regret it all
finally

    She didn't want to talk about it. She wanted me to see it, but she didn't want to talk about it. I thought there were plenty of reasons to discuss it. But I couldn't formulate a first question I was willing to ask and be willing to get an honest answer to. It took me a while to get over that stumbling block.

When Patricia dropped her honors strings class, it turned into a study hall. This became the time to do homework. All of a sudden, she'd come home without any schoolwork to do for tomorrow. I don't want to sound like the overbearing parent, but isn't part of the school experience learning how to manage and cope with homework? I recommended to Patricia that she take Mrs. Harris up on her offer to let her be a guidance helper during this study hall. She did. And it accomplished three things: It made the guidance office a familiar and comfortable place. Secondly, because one of the guidance helper duties is to be a messenger, it put her out into the school, sticking her head into different classrooms, delivering messages to teachers and students. Her school was so big that this was the only time she ever saw some of her friends. Finally, being a guidance helper meant she came home with lots of homework again. Patricia may not agree, but I choose to believe that this was a good thing.

∞

Patricia had a diagnosis of Bipolar Disorder, NOS. We're still not ready to talk about the NOS part, but we were trying to recognize the bipolar part in her. It's supposed to mean there are alternating times of depression and mania. Depression we saw. Sadness. Melancholy. Losing interest in friends and fun things. The mania was more elusive. We blamed the hopping up and down on one foot while spinning in a circle while smiling at the ceiling thing on the Prozac, so that didn't count. But we did see something else. By October, Patricia was getting more talkative. The less technical term might be diarrhea of the mouth. She'd start talking and wouldn't stop. She'd tell a story about school or friends. She'd smile. Clearly, she was enjoying herself. She went on and on. After a while, I'd start to worry. Because I knew what was next: A victim would conveniently present itself. Maybe a button on the computer didn't do what she wanted. Maybe her sister gave her a look. Maybe one of those juniors asked a stupid question in math class earlier that day. Something like, "What's an irrational number?" I knew what an irrational kid was. And like math, the result was always the same: She'd explode. Eventually. She'd shout. She'd rant. It had nothing to do with the earlier story. It just never happened unless there was an earlier story. This was completely out of character for Patricia. Other people acted like this. Never Patricia. Until now. And because the computer is an inanimate object, and because the math-class-junior was at football practice, it was usually Beth, her sister, who got to take the brunt of her anger. It was undeserved. This time.

That it was undeserved was not lost on Patricia either. She knew she wasn't handling things in the most appropriate way. It embarrassed her. It worried her. She went for a walk. She wondered how long it would take her parents to notice she was gone. She wondered where she would go if she kept walking. The problem was that I already had my copy of the poem with the answers to those questions. It scared me.

∞

There are four of us in the family. Six, actually, if you count the fish and the dog. This is supposed to be a story about Patricia. I've been trying to keep Beth, her younger sister, and Kate, my wife, out of it. Each played an important role in our journey, but to protect their privacy, I'm going to continue to leave them out as much as possible after this brief update. Here's why:

Kate had spent the previous year recovering from her stroke. She spent weeks in a rehabilitation hospital relearning how to walk. She spent months in physical therapy getting most of the strength back on one side of her body and (almost) straightening out her beautiful smile. Kate and I could talk about what was going on with Patricia, but after a few minutes, she changed the subject or went back to her television shows. Kate always had incredible insight into what was going on with Patricia. But her stamina hadn't returned enough for her to be completely involved.

Beth was trying to lead the life of a new middle-schooler during all of this. She had friends and basketball and soccer and gymnastics and dances and music lessons and sleepovers. Because Kate wasn't driving, I was chauffeur to the mall and all the other places sixth graders need to be. Despite all the time we were spending with Patricia, we worked very hard not to forget Beth. I spent a huge amount of time with her.

When Patricia was first hospitalized, we told Beth about the pills. We used the word "sad." Beth put those two together and had a pretty good picture of what was going on. She didn't understand it, but accepted it for what it was. Over the next several months, she did her best to be supportive. But as time went by, and as Patricia's behavior became more bizarre, Beth tired of it all. She got angrier and angrier. She wasn't always happy being the innocent victim for Patricia's next outburst. And I didn't blame her.

After the second hospitalization, we shared more and more with Beth. But the problem is that nothing made any sense. I could never find the words to describe what was going on with Patricia that would justify her behavior. If I had been able to do that, we would have known what to do about it. Sometimes Beth felt she was being left out of the loop, when in reality, she saw many things happening before I did. Ultimately, all we could do was find ways for Beth to vent.

That's all you get. Back to our story.

The one about Patricia. And school nurses. And guidance counselors. And others, too. Just not about Kate and Beth.

Please get over it. Because we are moving on without them.

∞

The school nurse has one role in life. The guidance counselor has another. There must be a line somewhere between the two. If the nurse just deals with medical issues and the guidance counselor deals with the trials and tribulations of being a student, where does sadness or feeling unsafe fall on the line? And whose job is it to teach an already fragile adolescent which is which? And whose job is it to make sure the adolescent still knows the answer when it matters most? Patricia would go see the nurse when she had a headache. She was having lot of headaches, so she saw the nurse lots of times. But she decided not to go to either one when she didn't feel safe in Latin class the day there was a substitute teacher filling in. Because neither one could have done anything anyway. Neither could I. Dr. Goodman wasn't having a whole lot of success either. Is that a reason to stop talking with us? I hope not.

∞

"Suicidal ideations" was another new phrase entering our vocabulary. It came up a lot. It means Patricia was spending time thinking about suicide. Patricia was clearly unhappy with how she was feeling. We'd been assured by everyone that asking would never "increase the likelihood" she would actually commit to suicide. It didn't mean she wouldn't, just that it wasn't any more likely than it already was that she would. When we asked Patricia, we always got us an honest answer. One we didn't want to hear.

Some kids use the threat of suicide as a tool. A weapon. Or a lever. To get their way. To make others miserable. Or for the rush associated with watching other's reaction to the threat. It's good for that. With Patricia, when she said she wanted to be dead, she wanted to be dead. We knew her well enough to know there wasn't any manipulation going on. Besides, telling us didn't win her anything. By the end of their second meeting with Patricia, all the professionals agreed with our assessment.

We also knew that anxiety was playing a part in Patricia's struggles. It was also a vicious circle that fed on itself. Her anxiety was keeping her from doing things she used to like to do. And getting home safe from things that didn't work out stoked the fires even more. Thinking about what others thought made it even worse.

∞

Shortly after Kate and I were married, our home phone started ringing off the hook. People were calling to schedule service appointments for their cars. It took a while to figure out that the local auto dealership had printed our phone number on the postcard they mail home saying your parts are in. Kate called the service department and explained the situation to the service rep. He said they'd had that number for years. It wasn't their problem. Click.

Not surprisingly, the calls didn't stop.

I called back and asked to speak to the general manager. He found one of the postcards. Sure enough, our number was there. "We'll take care of it," he said. The calls stopped for a couple of weeks, then started again. I wrote him a letter. The calls continued. I called again. "Nothing to worry about. We'll correct it." The calls stopped for a while, then started again. The final straw was when a police officer from the next town over woke up my sick wife from a delirious sleep and demanded to know what time she was open.

It took a letter to the president of General Motors to stop the calls. I explained that my wife and I were doing our best to be cordial, but I felt it wasn't a very smart business model to bet their customers on a system that had a stack of postcards with the wrong number on the shelf and relied on the mail clerk to remember to fix it every time before sending one out.

It seems like a stupid way to run a company. Or a life.

With Patricia, I spent a good deal of time worrying about what might set her off. What she was doing to keep busy. Who she was hanging out with. The words we used when we talked with her. Part of me wanted to protect her from the next thing that might make her anxious, but at the same time, I didn't want to deny her the childhood where you need to experience those feelings so you can learn to cope with what life throws at you. Still, I worried about what it might take for Patricia to snap and just end it all.

Her previous suicide attempts were planned. Thought about over time. She was telling us she was unhappy. She reported suicidal thoughts. That means some kind of planning was going on. The question was if, and when, she'd actually act on those plans. Patricia is smart. I had no question she could come up with a better way. One day, she told me she was regretting reading the article in the local paper about Brian's suicide. Now she was having thoughts about the method he chose. Quick and easy.

Ultimately, the computer at Patricia's school almost killed her. I'm convinced of it. Of all the things I was worried about, that wasn't on the list of possibilities. It never occurred to me to worry about systems. One day, a letter arrived in the mail from school saying that because Patricia had missed so many days, she would not be getting course credit for some of her classes.

Something must be wrong. She was getting straight A's. The hospital had a classroom. Patricia had done all the work the school asked her to do, so she had received credit for each day she was hospitalized. Her 504 Plan excused absences for counseling and medical appointments. But we'd done a pretty good job of keeping those outside of regular school hours. What could be wrong?

I called Brenda Harris. I could hear her jaw drop over the phone. There is a distinctive sound. You'll know it if you ever hear it. She checked. She told me that the computer automatically sends out these letters. But it shouldn't have sent that one. She's fine. Just ignore it. Although Brenda and I had decided not to tell Patricia about it, later that night, as Patricia and I were coming home from an emergency visit with Dr. Goodman, I was trying to make small talk with my unhappy child. I decided she needed to hear a funny story. So I told her about the letter. It was just the computer. *Nothing to worry about.*

The next day, one of her teachers handed her his copy of the letter. No explanation, just, "Here." This guy had a copy of Patricia's 504 Plan. He knew she was getting straight A's in his class. He knew she had already made up all the missing work. I don't know what he was thinking. He should have known better. Instead, he used his ninth-graders-are-old-enough-to-be-treated-like-adults blinders and gave her the letter.

I called Brenda again. I could hear her jaw drop. Again. Same sound. She checked. She told me the teacher should not have given that letter to Patricia. Never. Not under any circumstances. I knew that. I have no doubt that if I hadn't mentioned it to Patricia, she would have committed to suicide again. It turns out the school had a system that was betting my child's life that no one would give Patricia that letter. The computer never should have printed it out. I blame the system. Not the teacher. I began to question whether her school could keep her safe. By that time, I was beginning to believe they had some responsibility to try.

∞

Patricia was pretty good at reporting how she was feeling, but her timing wasn't always good. Feeling miserable and feeling anxious were a part of daily life. Unfortunately, they were also just one more item to put on the list of things to prioritize. And they didn't always end up in the right spot on the list.

One day, she went off to school. Went to class. And thought about suicide. She considered going to the guidance office to call home to let me know, but she decided not to. Her next class was guidance helper. Not as stressful as the previous class. She felt better. So she didn't say anything to Mrs. Harris. Why should she? After school that day, I picked her up at the end of the road. Patricia was startled I was there. "Why are you here?" *We need to get to your appointment with Deb on time.* "Oh."

After Patricia's session, I had one of my confused-parent talks with Deb. I was trying to understand just how much I should be in

Patricia's face asking her how she is feeling. Deb said Patricia is better. That she can identify problems and talk about them. That I should keep asking, but back off when Patricia asks me to.

That night, as sometimes happened, Patricia had a fight with Beth. At the height of it, Patricia announced, "Well, I'll just leave," and walked out of the house. That had never happened before. I gave her a while, and then went outside to find her. I did. Crying. "I was going to run, but I didn't know where to go."

She talked about earlier in the day. She decided not to tell me or Deb how she was feeling because she didn't want to end up in the hospital again. "But I want you to know about how I'm feeling before I'm dead." "Now I'm in over my head. Deb won't trust me or believe me when I say I'm OK." "I'm back to square two because no one is going to trust me."

She was right.

∞

For someone so unstable and trying so hard to keep it together, her classmates still needed her. Sometimes to their detriment. I got a call from Mrs. Harris. Patricia had come to see her in a panic. History had been tough. Her classmates had been difficult. Apparently they weren't paying attention enough to meet Patricia's high standards. She started getting anxious. Then came science. When her tablemates asked her for the lab data they all should have been collecting on their own papers, she started getting worse. Parabolically.

When they asked her for the data a second time, she snapped at them, said something about the need to pay attention, and fled to the restroom. She told me later that she lamented to the bathroom mirror, "They don't care about me. No one cares about me." She worried if she went back to class and came home on the bus, that she wouldn't say anything to anybody about this. So she went to guidance and called home. I picked her up. She improved dramatically. She went to see Deb for her regular session, came home, and slept great. In the morning, she emailed an apology to her teacher and Mrs. Harris, went off to school and had a great day. Talking with Mrs. Harris later, we decided the teacher never noticed that Patricia did something that required an apology. And we speculated her tablemates never took notice of Patricia's outburst. Regular kids have hissy fits now and then. It's normal. But not for Patricia.

∞

Those characters were back. They'd been around now and then for several months. Every time they showed up, we'd learn a little bit more about them. They would disappear for a while after a medication change, but they always came back. Patricia usually didn't notice unless asked. Until Kevin started mouthing off.

Kevin is one of the imaginary characters. And Kevin started talking *to* Patricia: "Look at those cuts on your wrists."

Patricia hadn't been cutting for months. There weren't any cuts on her wrists. Besides, when she did cut, she cut her ankles. Kevin didn't know what he was talking about. But that didn't silence him:

"What are you doing here? You died yesterday."

Uh-oh. This isn't good.

∞

More trouble at school. One of her science classmates ruined the graph. Spilled something on it. It was up to Patricia to fix it. Bullheaded Patricia had a plan: She was going to make a new one in Excel®. But she wasn't good enough at it to be able to make a graph. That reality didn't matter. She still needed to make a new one. In Excel®. I asked if she could just clean off the old graph? "No." I wondered if she might just draw one? "No." She worked herself up into a tizzy. Burst into tears. And went to bed.

The next morning before school, I taught her how to make a graph. I'm not sure if that was the right thing to do, but it solved the problem. And gave her a new life-skill.

∞

Medicine wasn't helping. Everything Dr. Goodman tried seemed to make things worse. One day, he handed me a piece of paper. It had one word on it: "Clozapine." He asked us to check it out and think about it. Clozapine is a powerful antipsychotic drug. According to Dr. Goodman, it has a proven track record of protecting against suicide. It also has some of those pesky side-effects: Death is the important one. But it doesn't usually happen, because all you need to do is get a blood test. Every week for six months. Every other week for another six months. Then every 28 days. Forever.

Clozapine is a big deal. This is a medicine you really don't want to be on. Unless you need to be.

To help us with our decision, Dr. Goodman asked us to go see the new child psychiatrist in his practice, Dr. Washburn, for a second opinion. The timing of this was either convenient or conspired: Dr. Goodman was going on vacation next month for three weeks. Dr. Washburn would cover while he was gone. We were lucky to make it one week between appointments with Dr. Goodman. We'd never made it anywhere near three.

We'd never been to a second opinion before, so I didn't know what to expect. I dusted off my notes. You remember the ones: Kate's stroke, smart kid, contemplative, wise beyond her years, creative, music, books, movies, Brian, Holocaust unit, friends, Destination Imagination, sensitive, fragile. We didn't need any of it. We were in and out of his office in 10 minutes. He glanced at her chart, asked a couple of questions, and announced it was way too soon to be considering Clozapine. He said to try Depakote. Or Tegretol. More Lithium. Or Risperdal.

Two days later, at the last minute, Deb called and cancelled her session with Patricia. We really liked Deb, but her timing was poor. It seemed as if she only cancelled on the really bad days. Or maybe every day was bad. That could also explain the pattern. Patricia was agitated and went off to bed early. I followed, trying to make small talk. "Leave me alone." *What should we do?* "I don't know ... if I did, I'd be doing it."

This was an important answer to a really stupid question.

I always thought that if we could talk about it, we could figure out what to do. You remember, the scientific method.

I was too dumb to leave, so I persisted: "Who are you mad at? Me? Mom? Beth?"

"Life."

So I made her take a shower and help me wash the dishes. She did. And improved dramatically.

$$- \overset{54}{\underset{107}{\bigcirc}} + \boxed{C110}$$

Trouble Staying in School

Destination Imagination was consuming more and more time. The tournament was approaching fast. For months, Patricia's team had been building medieval castles, thatching the roofs of cardboard huts, and sewing costumes. The script and songs were coming along fine—something about a knight who is scared of his own shadow. Patricia had an important part: She would play the traveling minstrel. She'd set the stage, play some period music she wrote for the viola, and serve as narrator.

Meetings, which used to be once a week for two hours, were now every day. And every night. And for just as long as possible. It was winter, so a snow day gave them an extra eight hours to meet. There were sleepovers—yes—Patricia could still do those—but her anxiety was building day by day. So was mine. She came home from one overnight and said, "Thanks for letting me sleep over last night. If I was at home, I think I would have cut." I'm glad this wasn't part of the conversation when I agreed to let her go.

At another meeting, they were working on their story line. Patricia had an idea, but lost it. Someone asked for her opinion. She didn't know what to say. So she burst into tears. And fled to the bathroom. She called me. "What should I do?" *I don't know;* but I couldn't say that. We agreed that she'd wash her face, work up her courage, go back to her meeting, and try again. She went back and made it through the meeting. She came home pleased. I began to wonder what she was pleased about. Being an important contributor to her team? Or making it through the meeting? Which was more important to her? How about to her teammates?

During the few minutes we spent together at home or in the car, our conversations became more ominous.

"I feel safe, but I don't want to be alive.

"Utter confusion.

"It's bugging me ... not knowing what's wrong. Not being able to describe what I'm feeling."

The problem with this statement is that Patricia was doing a great job of describing how miserable she was. It was no secret. She seemed to be sharing perfectly well that something was wrong. It turns out there is a difference between knowing something is wrong and knowing what is wrong. Because you can't begin to think about fixing it until you know what actually is wrong.

There was no school the Friday before Saturday's DI tournament. Professional Development Day for the teachers. Maybe they were off learning not to give the kid with a 504 Plan a copy of the letter from the misinformed computer saying she's flunking out of school. Whatever the teachers were doing gave Patricia's team an extra 24 hours to get ready for the tournament. There was a sleepover on Thursday and a meeting all day Friday.

At two o'clock Friday, I got a call from Patricia: Full blown panic attack. "Come get me." I did. Tears. Benadryl. Hot shower. *Can you go back?* "Not yet." To bed.

At four o'clock, Patricia got out of bed, dressed, and went back to her meeting. She managed to tell her teammates—her friends— that she wasn't able to perform her part tomorrow. They accepted the reality. And because DI is DI, and because DI means figure it out, they figured it out. As a team. Their team only had six members that year. The rules allowed a maximum of seven. They called James. He'd been on the team last year, but had dropped out. He showed up. At six o'clock. With a shower curtain. They made it into a toga. They spent their last few hours before tournament day splitting Patricia's part in two. The talking part. And the musician part.

The next day, James played the part of narrator. Brilliantly. He set the scene. And told the story of the fraidy-cat knight as he traveled from the village with the thatched roofed huts to the glorious castle. Patricia played her viola—the traveling minstrel. Their team came in second place—just where they would have come in even if they were 10 times better. The winning team was a bunch of barbershop pirates from Monson with a handmade Broadway-quality sailing ship and Toni-Award-winning original music—the same team who beat them the year before. And the year before that.

James won a special Spirit of DI Award. A Spirit of Discovery and Imagination Award is given to those rare teams or individuals who go out of their way to help others, making sacrifices not for themselves, but to give something to someone else. He deserved it.

After the tournament was over, there was a huge sigh of relief. It was as if a heavy weight had been lifted. You could see it in Patricia's face. In her demeanor. She smiled. We'd been missing that. She talked about looking forward to DI next year.

The turnaround lasted one day.

On Monday, after school, in the car, on the way to see Dr. Washburn, I asked Patricia what she was going to say to him.

"If I could find the antifreeze, I will kill myself today." *Uh-oh.*

This is not the kind of response I was expecting or wanted to hear. I was hoping Patricia would spend a few minutes in the car gathering her thoughts for the doctor so we could make good use of our short time with him. I didn't want her to be unclear or uncertain about her feelings. She didn't disappoint. She was very clear and very concise. That's my kid.

There isn't anything in the parenting manual we got from the hospital the day Patricia was born about how the responsible adult is supposed to react to such a comment. I grabbed the wheel a little tighter, focused my eyes ahead on the road, and tried my best to keep my expression neutral. Driving into a tree or bursting into tears were two other possibilities.

Thank you for telling me.

Some children make outlandish statements to get attention. They don't mean what they say. Patricia had plenty of attention. It wasn't making her any better, but she didn't need to say something like that to get people to notice she was feeling awful. But it might have been what she needed to say to get herself back into the hospital. So someone else could try again to make her feel better.

It took me a couple of days, but I checked the Internet history logs on Patricia's computer. She had been exploring different suicide methods for about two weeks. She'd chosen antifreeze among several possibilities. She'd done extensive research.

Our meeting with Dr. Washburn was short. He sent us off to East Side Emergency Mental Health. He told Patricia she needed a major medication change. And that it should take place in the hospital. Where she would be safe.

Patricia ended up in the hospital again. No surprise. But still, it took 14 hours to make it there. The first 10 were spent waiting for an evaluation. The next three were spent with East Side EMH calling the Children's Psychiatric Unit at Patriot Medical and telling them Patricia needed to go there. Patriot Medical kept saying they didn't have any room. But because they don't discharge kids in the middle of the night, somebody must have worn someone else down, because by three a.m., space magically opened up. Patricia went and slept in the quiet room.

The social worker was back from maternity leave. This meant we needed to bring a new person up to speed on Patricia's history and current status. It also complicated things. Now we had a social worker, a psychologist, a psychiatrist, the head nurse, and the clinical staff. I still didn't know what a social worker does. Adding another person just further reduced the chances of directing today's question to the right person.

What didn't change was the immediate realization that the hospital wanted her out of there. They had no interest in considering any kind of significant medication change. Stabilize. Send home. But once again, Patricia foiled their plans: She didn't stabilize. She didn't get better. She didn't calm down. She was angry at the hospital. For several reasons:

Patricia was angry because she had been in the room when Dr. Washburn said she needed a major medication change. And it should take place in the hospital. Why weren't they doing anything? Because their job is to stabilize. And send home. That's why.

Patricia was also angry that they still wouldn't help her with her safety plan. "Best we've ever seen." But clearly there was something wrong with it.

Let's take a look.

Patricia's Safety Plan	
Distance from Suicide	**Coping Techniques**
Bad Mood	Make a Smoothie Knit/Crochet Bike Ride, Jump Rope Go to Pool/Library
Feelings of Worthlessness/ Hopelessness	Take Care of Dog Brush Teeth Make a Smoothie/Hot Chocolate Knit/Crochet Bike Ride, Jump Rope Go to Pool/Library
Thinking of Cutting	Go for Walk Knit/Crochet Bike Ride, Jump Rope Go to Pool/Library
Cutting	Get Out of the House – Go to: The Pool/Library A Friend's House Schoolyard Friendly's for Ice Cream McDonald's for Fries/Milkshake Dunkin Donuts for Donut
Vague Thoughts of Suicide	Call friend
Plan of Suicide	Talk to Trusted Adult Dad Mom Lois, Eric Deb Aunt Ann Grandmother
Suicide	Call 911 or Go to ER

Can you see the problem? It's there. This plan was developed during Patricia's first hospitalization. It took until the third one to figure out how it is dangerously flawed. Patricia knew something was wrong with it. She asked the hospital to help her fix it. Twice, they told her it was the best safety plan they had ever seen. I wonder if they ever looked at it? Sure, it has lots of creative ideas. But it's supposed to be a safety plan.

The problem with this plan is that as Patricia gets closer and closer to suicide, she's moving farther and farther away from people who can help. Bad mood—smoothie. That happens in the kitchen. Feeling worthless—jump rope or bike ride. That's outside. Thinking of cutting—go for a walk. And what? Obsess about wanting to cut? Alone. Away from home. Actually cutting—swing on swings at school. That's a half hour walk from home. Plenty of time to think about where and how to cut. It's not until there is an actual plan for suicide that talking to someone even comes up.

They changed the safety plan.

Patricia was also angry that Dr. Chase, the psychologist, still wasn't attending groups. The social worker was back. So why couldn't he be running the groups again? She knew he did a better job than the recreational staff. He was a trained psychologist. They were trained babysitters. She wondered what she was even doing in the hospital. She asked. They said she was there to keep her safe and help plan for going home. But that's not why she went to the hospital. She went there for a major medication change.

∞

A couple of days into this hospitalization, when it became clear to the hospital staff that Patricia was not improving, I got a call from the hospital psychiatrist saying she wanted to start Patricia on Celexa, another antidepressant. We'd had some experience with one of those. Remember Prozac? That's the one that came with its own roadmap to suicide. I made two phone calls. The first went to Dr. Washburn. I left a message asking him to give me a call. The other went to Dr. Goodman. I knew he was leaving for his vacation later that day, but I decided to leave a message for him anyway. My question for both of them was whether they had an opinion about starting Patricia on Celexa.

Incredibly, Dr. Washburn called me back almost immediately. He was blunt and to the point: He said Celexa was an SSRI and anyone who prescribed one for Patricia after her reaction to Prozac was an idiot.

I got into my car and started driving to Patriot Medical. I was tooling down the Massachusetts Turnpike, practicing my speech for the psychiatrist, trying to get the words just right for when I would tell her that "only an idiot would prescribe Patricia Celexa," when Dr. Goodman called. He hadn't left yet. I shared my conversation with Dr. Washburn.

He thought for a moment, and then said, "It is important to respect the opinions of professionals and Patricia might be a good candidate for Celexa." Celexa won.

Over the next few days, I watched Patricia experience many of the same side-effects she had on Prozac. We got another checklist and started keeping score. Jumping up and down; while twirling in a circle; while talking a mile a minute. Check. Check. Check.

Every day, I'd visit Patricia and we'd mark something else off the list. I asked her if she'd kept the hospital staff informed about how she was doing. She expressed great frustration in not being able to get them to listen to all of her miserable side-effects. I found myself leaving the hospital, firing up the Bluetooth headset on my cellphone, and calling the nursing station to let them know the latest gossip about their patient. Ultimately, this behavior won me a special notation on the discharge paperwork: "The anxious father." Of course I was anxious. Who wouldn't be?

I wear it like a badge of honor.

Although the hospital wasn't listening, Patricia had lots to say. This was the first time she seemed to be aware of how badly she was feeling and had a genuine interest in making things better. She started asking questions: "What am I working on here?" And started making statements: "I don't want to spend the rest of my life coping with these feelings." I liked the first statement. I worried about the second one.

Communicating exactly what was going on inside Patricia turned out to be a challenging, convoluted problem. She didn't really know what was right with her and what was wrong. Putting it into words was impossible. And getting people to understand just how miserable she was feeling was counterproductive. Every time she stopped talking about wanting to kill herself long enough to describe the feelings that were driving her to want to kill herself, everyone remarked on how well she was doing. Being able to describe why you want to be dead doesn't make you better. It just demonstrates that your logic is sound.

I showed up at the hospital with two composition books. Patricia and I sat quietly at the end of her bed. I gave them to her and said I thought she should write a book. One composition book was for stories about how she feels. The other was for stories of happier times. It was very clear Patricia needed to spend time trying to understand what was going on, but it was also clear that her patience and stamina were strained by experiencing those same feelings. Ultimately, she wrote quite a bit. Poetry was her way.

As the Celexa kicked in, we started to see mania again. We had the hopping around, but there were racing thoughts, too: "Like fish in a net with holes too big so they never got caught enough to know what they are about." Who needs to know about this? What are they going to do about it? Like the fish, Patricia didn't understand enough to know what it was all about.

Then she got happy. Too happy. She needed to leave group. Because she was too happy. This didn't make a lot of sense. When you haven't been happy in a while, apparently being happy is a problem. It's just too much. But luckily, this is something you *can* practice. Practice feeling good. After a while you can get used to it. You get to spend time not being sad. It's work. But it's not that bad.

∞

Part of the hospital deal is to get blood tests now and then. They need to be sure they aren't killing you with all those drugs. In the process of procuring a blood sample, things don't always go well. Sometimes the phlebotomist, another new word, had a little trouble finding a vein. Maybe it took a couple of tries, or maybe she just used the needle like a divining rod, inside the arm, fishing for something red. One day, Patricia looked at her arm, smiled, and commented, "My blood-work bruise looks like a bipolar-awareness ribbon." Both are green. Did you catch the part about the smile?

∞

Despite everything else going wrong, one thing was going right. Something was happening. Patricia was getting better. She felt better. She looked better. Her anxiety was abating. After yet another 10-day hospital stay, they called me up and told me to come get her.

Being discharged from the hospital is like graduating from Motel 6. Get your stuff together and get out of here. Not a lot of pomp and circumstance. The last step is to meet with a nurse, get all the new prescriptions, and sign the discharge paperwork.

But I couldn't read the doctor's handwriting. By this time, I knew that without my signature, my kid wasn't going home. And I decided we weren't leaving until I knew what everything said. I asked the nurse what this word was. She didn't know. She went to ask the doctor. Then I asked what that word was. She didn't know. She went to ask the doctor. And so on. Until the psychiatrist finally just came out to talk with me. I asked what that word and these others were. She told me.

When I was satisfied and prepared to take Patricia home, I started to thank her for all she'd done for us. But instead of shaking hands and going our separate ways, she said, "Not so fast. You started this. I'm going to tell you what I think." She spent the next five minutes explaining what it all meant. She went through every part of the discharge paperwork and talked about Patricia's current status. As she spoke, she even changed Patricia's diagnosis. She said Patricia's anxiety was far more debilitating than her bipolar symptoms and we should be concentrating our efforts on anxiety.

I had been trying to get useful information from her for 10 days. Ultimately, I got it because I was unwilling to take Patricia home without being able to read her handwriting. Those few minutes with the psychiatrist were some of the best minutes I've ever had with a doctor. Any doctor. She told me what she thought. And she told me what we should be working on. Isn't that what medicine is supposed to be about?

Patricia's diagnosis changed today. It now is:
Bipolar Disorder, NOS
Mood Disorder, NOS
Anxiety Disorder, NOS.

∞

Unfortunately, getting better is different than being better. And unless you continue to get better, you never really get any closer to actually being better. Patricia was ready to come home from the hospital. She'd had enough of them. They'd had enough of her. But that didn't mean the anxiety was gone.

Returning to "normal" now had a couple of extra steps. We checked in with Dr. Washburn and Deb. There was a meeting at school. We tweaked the 504 Plan to include a weekly meeting with the guidance counselor. This was interesting because, on one hand, the school finally acknowledged that everything really wasn't fine and Patricia needed to be checking in with someone at school. But on the other hand, Patricia was already accessing her guidance counselor, sometimes many times each day, so maybe this line was really a tactic to reduce the frequency of their visits and that Patricia should be spending more time in class.

Catching up at school wasn't a big problem. Patricia had managed to do all the work her teachers had sent.

Catching up with friends was another important step. Patricia reconnected with her Destination Imagination team. They spent a Saturday going to the state tournament to watch Monson, the team that had beat them a few weeks earlier, secure their first-place medals so they could go on to Global Finals, the last competition of the year where all the best teams in the world get together at the University of Tennessee in Knoxville.

Sure, her team welcomed her back, but remember, she wasn't all better. I saw things. I'm sure her friends did too. I drove her to the state tournament to meet up with her teammates that day. To finance her lunch, I handed her a few one-dollar bills. To make sure she had enough, I asked her to count them. She couldn't. Huh? She tried a couple of times, and then handed them back to me. It was bizarre. Patricia used to be able to count.

Two days later, Patricia was sitting at home at her computer doing her homework. Clearly, she was agitated about something. She told me, "My thoughts are spinning." I asked her to write me an email to describe how she felt. She glared at me for a second, then turned back to her computer and started typing. Clickety clack. Clickety clack. Bang. Bang. Bang. CLICKETY CLACK. BANG. BANG. BANG.

I don't know why, but I knew those bangs were the backspace key. It was obvious. She'd be typing a mile a minute, then Bang. Bang. Bang. A couple of minutes later, quiet descended over the house. A moment after that, this showed up in my email inbox:

BY EMAIL
From: Patricia
To: Dad
Subject:

My thoughts are turning. Like a merry-go-round. A merry-go-round full of kids, spinning faster and faster every second. I'm trying to do my homework. I can see it there, in front of me, but there's nothing I can do in it. I know that the thought that gives me the ability to do this worksheet is somewhere on this merry-go-round, hidden within one of those kids. It seems like there are hundreds of others, and every time I reach and grab for the right kid another one ends up in my grasp. Soon I'm so preoccupied with how I have the wrong kid that I forget who I'm looking for. I look down at my books and am reminded who and what I'm trying to grab and start the futile task all over again. My dad says I'm typing fast and am getting aggravated but all I can focus on is how hard I'm tapping the keys and how much harder I tap the 'backspace' key than the other ones. Then I forget that and start thinking about something else, only to be reminded of all the mistakes in what I'm typing a second later. I want to give up on thinking at all, just go to sleep. Somehow I know that I have to stand and face this; keep hitting the backspace key, keep grabbing for that kid, keep forgetting what I was trying to do a second ago. Then I forget… Then I remember… Then I forget.
—Patricia

Notice there isn't one typo.

Patricia had another bad day. She and Beth fought over the shower. I don't know why, we have two. The next day, she admitted to cutting again the night before. "Just a little blood. What's the big deal?" "But I don't want to get caught because I'll never be trusted again."

Deb said the characters were present.

Patricia developed a kind of cough. She'd clear her throat. Just once. Three or four times per minute. All day long. Every day. Months later, when one of Patricia's classmates made a comment about it, the cough disappeared. And it didn't come back.

I called the psychiatrist at Patriot Medical. I was trying to get her to write the discharge summary for Patricia's hospitalization. It still wasn't done. Incredibly, she came to the phone. And said, "Deep down inside, Patricia is not that sick." What she didn't tell me was how to integrate that comment into our daily routine.

Dr. Goodman was expected back from vacation. Because it worked so well last time, we started making a list of things to talk about at our next meeting. "I have a fear of dropping out of school." "I'm afraid to think." "I fear that people can read my thoughts." "I'm tired in the morning." "My head throbs." "My ears are ringing." "I'm dizzy in class." When he came back, we gave him a copy of the hospital paperwork and shared our list of complaints. He said he was still thinking about Clozapine and we should get a second opinion from McLean, or Children's, or Mass General, three of the top hospitals in Boston.

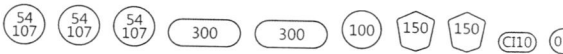

— ⊙ + ③

Second Opinion

We had experience getting a second opinion. Dr. Washburn had done one for us the month before. I was still uncertain about this Celexa business and wanted to get a fresh opinion on that too while we investigated Clozapine. My goal was to have this done in two weeks, in time for our next appointment with Dr. Goodman. *Boy, am I stupid.*

I called McLean Hospital. I knew about them. They were famous for their breakthrough research into bipolar disorder. One of my favorite musicians spent much of his childhood in their residential program. At parent support groups, I was starting to meet parents of children who were getting real help there. I called. They said they don't do second opinions anymore. They told me to call Dr. Sharon Barnes's office at the Child and Adolescent Unit at Mystic Valley Healthcare. I called them. They promised to talk with Dr. Barnes about a consult and get back to me within a week. OK. But I was still hoping get something in time for our meeting with Dr. Goodman.

I called Children's Hospital. They said no. Well, actually, they said they were booked solid for four months, they weren't making any more appointments, and I should go elsewhere.

Then I called Mass General. They said sure. All I needed to do was switch Patricia's primary care physician from her doctor in Worcester, seven miles from home, to one of their doctors, an additional 50 miles of brutal traffic and impossible parking away. I sometimes wonder if the lady I was talking to was serious, or if she just hangs up the phone and bursts out laughing every time a desperate parent like me calls.

Mystic Valley Healthcare called back to say that Dr. Barnes agreed to meet with Patricia. Great! The way it would work is we'd first meet with Leslie Steiner, one of Dr. Barnes's associates. That would happen in about a month. She'd talk with Patricia. A couple of weeks later, we'd meet with Dr. Barnes. In the meantime, we were supposed to email them a history of where we were. Next, we'd sign some release of information forms so they could talk with Dr. Goodman, Deb, the school, and DMH. So much for surprising Dr. Goodman with a thoughtful second opinion at our meeting next week. So much for a five minute second opinion like we'd had with the other doctor. This was starting to seem real. It was beginning to look like we had finally found someone who could actually help. I made the appointment.

∞

It was time for me to get organized. This had been going on long enough. I had little scraps of paper filling up my pockets and a couple of 3″ x 5″ spiral-bound notebooks filled with snippets of everything that had happened during the last year. We had our Collaborative Assessment report. I had my list. Kate's stroke, smart kid, and so on. I still hadn't figured out which of those things were important. And so much had happened in the last year to add to our story. I hadn't committed any of this, officially, to paper. It was time.

I come from a printing background. Somehow that makes me understand the importance of a good letter. On nice stationery. By email? Sure, I can do that. I already had an email template in a readable font with my name, address and contact information. That would be the delivery vehicle for one multi-page PDF attachment including a cover letter, detailed history and various other attachments. I added my email address to my most conservative personal letterhead template, called my sister to find out what to say, and started typing.

First we need a cover letter. Never more than one page. To introduce all the people in our drama, list everything included in the packet, and most importantly, ask for something.

Bob Larsted
A Quiet Street · Holden, Massachusetts 01520
508 555-0196 · bob@boblarsted.com

Leslie Steiner
Mystic Valley Healthcare

Dear Leslie,

Enclosed is background information for our May 30th 11:00 a.m. appointment regarding Patricia. We, Patricia's parents, together with her psychiatrist and psychologist, are seeking consultation around medication and treatment planning.

After a relatively uneventful childhood, Patricia's mental health has dramatically deteriorated in the past year. The current medication regime and various support services are not working to stabilize her or to return Patricia to a positive life course.

Questions:

Medication: Current regime does not stabilize Patricia's mood and does not eliminate auditory hallucinations, suicidal ideation, cutting, or panic attacks. It does successfully get Patricia to sleep, but no longer gives her restorative sleep. Patricia's psychiatrist has asked us to consider Clozapine. Do you have recommendations regarding any aspects of these medications?

Other Treatment Options: Do you have suggestions for supports that would be helpful if Patricia has another episode of significant decompensation? Do you have suggestions for other supports?

Parental Support: We, as parents, are new to this. Do you have advice on how to anticipate and manage mood shifts and "incidents" as they occur?

We look forward to our appointment on May 30.

Sincerely,
Patricia's Father

My sister wrote most of this. It's not my words. They are hers. I don't talk like that. It's too clinical. However, it makes sense.

∞

There is a hamburger joint near us. All they sell is hamburgers. But I didn't used to be able to eat there. The problem is the menu. There isn't one hamburger on it. The kid behind the register wears a bright orange bandana and a plastic 10-gallon hat. The menu consists of things like "The Yee Haw," "The Pardner," and "The Feedbag." As I make my way to the head of the line and the guy in front of me orders his "Whippersnapper" with extra "Loco Sauce," I have to leave. All I want is a cheeseburger with lettuce, tomato, and ketchup. It's called "The Roundup." But I can't say that.

If I tried to order a cheeseburger with lettuce, tomato, and ketchup, time would stop. Someone in the back would turn off the hootenanny music; all the customers would turn their heads and stare at me. The guy behind the register would glare—his braces just barely visible behind his quivering lip, looking like barbed wire—and he would say, "Huh?" This guy would have no idea what I was talking about. Because they don't sell cheeseburgers. They sell "The Roundup." And if you want a cheeseburger with lettuce, tomato, and ketchup, you need to order "The Roundup."

My problem is I can't bring myself to use their lingo. In the case of the cheeseburger, it's stupid and embarrassing. In the case of what's going on with my child, it's frightening. And embarrassing. As I looked at that cover letter and settled down to write Patricia's history for Dr. Barnes, I started to change. I could write about "taking some pills" and "characters." But the problem is that no one knows what it means except for me. "Auditory hallucinations" and "suicidal ideation" mean things. You can talk about them and do things. "Significant decompensation" are two words that perfectly describe everything we'd gone through in the past year. Anything else would be 10 pages—or 100—like we're at now. In order to keep the cover letter to one page and to ask for something that might actually help, I knew my vocabulary needed to be updated to what the guy behind the counter would understand. It didn't make it any less embarrassing, but we really needed help. We needed advice on how to help Patricia return to "a positive life course."

Writing the history was brutal. For the first time ever, all the terrible things that had been going on for the past year were written down in one place. It was three and a half pages long. Like any good resume, there were several carefully labeled sections:

Patricia's History

- ☐ *Name, Date of Birth, Age.*
- ☐ *Address, Phone Number, Dad's Cell Phone Number.*
- ☐ *Current Diagnosis.*
- ☐ *Current Medications and Dosages.*
- ☐ *Discontinued Medications.*
- ☐ *Current Services.*
- ☐ *Family Members, along with significant medical and mental health history.*
- ☐ *Patricia's Medical and Developmental History.*
- ☐ *School Information.*
- ☐ *Friend and Passions.*
- ☐ *And a History of what had been going on. Everything, including auditory hallucinations, sleep, cutting, suicide attempts, hospitalizations, a teen suicide in town, reactions and side-effects for each of the discontinued and current medications, the new cough. I included selected quotations from Patricia relating to each of these items.*
- ☐ *Finally, Unresolved Issues. For us, this meant: "Auditory hallucinations, suicidal ideations, anxiety, exhausted during the day (even after 9 hours of sleep), paranoia, shaking, twitching (particularly the knee), headaches, and cough.*

I knew that was a long list, but I had no idea what to leave out. So everything stayed.

One more thing. To make this the history of a real person and not just of the next kid in a long list of people to see today, I added Patricia's picture at the top of the page. Just a small copy of her school picture stuck up there in the corner.

The cover letter was done. Page one. The history was done. Pages two through five. Page six was a copy of Patricia's most recent report card. Page seven was the accommodations page from her 504 Plan. Page eight finished it off with copies of her "Thoughts are Turning" email and this note, something she handed me one particularly tough day. Something else I didn't know how to react to:

~~Something's wrong.~~ Something's not right. I think it's been going on all day, maybe longer. Everything's dark again, like wearing glasses. I've been distracted ... in class, at lunch, trying to document this ... etc. I think I'm feeling a connection with everything ... being apologetic to my shoelace for having it tied too tight, feeling like I'm wearing Nathan's sunglasses and not him which is why it's so dark, feeling misunderstood as the piece of gravel casts away to the side of the street ... then I feel guilty for having more of a choice than my shoelace and not taking the chance (which I may or may not deserve) to untie myself. So ... the worst part is the guilt, which comes out of nowhere, telling me to stop complaining about my problems and either fix them or deal with them because I have the ability to. Then part of me says 'Can I really fix it?' and the other part says 'shut up.' I just ... feel like I need to do something a certain way, like writing this so small.
So, sorry. I just can't help it.
—Patricia

I emailed everything off to Dr. Barnes's office. I called them the next day to be sure they would have it before our meeting with Leslie. They did. It was exactly what they were looking for. Great.

We had an appointment with Deb coming up. I wanted to get her feedback to make sure we hadn't left out anything significant. To give her a chance to look at it before Patricia's appointment, I printed out copies of everything, wrote a quick note, put it all in a flat envelope with her name printed in big letters on the front and drove it down to her office. I gave it the receptionist and asked her to please give it to Deb so she'd have it before our meeting the next day. She promised she would.

By now, you must know what's coming. I didn't have a clue. We went to see Deb. "What envelope?" *Uh, the one I dropped off for you yesterday.* "What was in it?" We never got Deb's input.

But of course it didn't really matter because you must know what's coming next, too. And again, I still didn't have a clue. We showed up at our appointment with Leslie Steiner. "What history?" *The one I emailed to your office.* "What did it say?" *Uh.*

Despite everything, our meeting with Leslie was wonderful. She found the history and all the other papers. She spent a long time with Patricia. And then nearly as long with Patricia and Kate and me. Patricia did a great job of answering her questions. We'd heard many of them before. "Do you hear voices?" *No.* "Do you see things other people don't see?" *No.* "Is anyone commanding you to do something?" *No.* "Have you been feeling anxious or panicky?" *Yes.* "Do you think people are watching you?" *Yes.* "Do you think others can control your thoughts?" *Probably not.* "Do you think you can control other's thoughts?" *Maybe.*

Notice the answer to the "Do you hear voices?" questions was still "No." Leslie and Patricia talked about these characters. Leslie probed. Finally she asked Patricia how often the characters are present and what they talk about. Patricia replied, "Well, right now, they are talking about spontaneous combustion."

I think I saw Leslie flinch, but she kept her composure.

Apparently, during our entire meeting that day, the car ride there, during breakfast that morning, the day before, and probably for weeks before that, these characters had been talking to Patricia about everything around her bursting into flames. But she still couldn't identify them as voices. They told her stories. They talked to her. But she couldn't identify them as voices. They were her imaginary friends. Gone bad.

They were voices.

We came back in a couple of weeks and met with Leslie and Dr. Barnes. They spent lots more time with Patricia. When they were done, Dr. Barnes handed me a report for Dr. Goodman. It was three pages long. You know I had a hard time writing Patricia's history. I had an even harder time reading Dr. Barnes's report.

Here we had doctor talking to doctor in brutal, clinical terms. It confirmed Patricia was having auditory, tactile, and olfactory hallucinations. There were voices. She could feel things that weren't there. And she could smell things that weren't there. There were at least three voices telling her stories. One voice was diabolical. Another was capable of reading her mind. One of several recurring subjects was spontaneous combustion. It acknowledged Patricia's bizarre dreams.

It talked about the Celexa. Dr. Barnes didn't like it. It really wasn't doing anything to lift the depression. Patricia told Dr. Barnes, "Ever since I started on it, I feel like I can sharpen pencils with my mind." But except for a couple of times she was really, really happy, most of the time she felt dark and empty. She said that during her previous suicide attempts, she wanted to die and was sorry she had not succeeded.

Ugh.

It had a long list of recommendations. Finally, something to do. A sleep deprived EEG, and MRI. All kinds of blood tests. Just to make sure there isn't some other reason for Patricia's symptoms. Get rid of the Celexa. Slowly. Neuropsychological and projective testing. But not until she's stable. (I could never have guessed how long that might be.) Continued therapy.

Leslie and Dr. Barnes agreed that Patricia needed a "med-wash." And it should happen at McLean Hospital. A "med-wash" is where you slowly and carefully wean off one medicine or medicines before starting slowly on something else. It's supposed to minimize a whole different collection of side-effects. For Patricia and the medicines she was taking, deadly seizures and suicide were two of the more important ones.

Dr. Barnes recommended Clozapine as the replacement drug. It turns out she knows quite a bit about it. She was scheduled to give a talk to present her research findings to the medical community later that week. Her clinical trials demonstrated that Clozapine, despite its sinister reputation, is actually a safe and effective protection against suicide in adolescents. Unfortunately, Patricia needed it. Dr. Barnes told us we had two treatment plans to choose from: Start Patricia on Risperdal, which won't work, or, start her on Clozapine, which will.

Patricia's diagnosis changed today. It now is:
Schizoaffective Disorder.

"Schizoaffective Disorder." But there was another phrase in the report: "Treatment Refractory." It means that it's treatment resistant. It means medications haven't worked. It means it might not be that easy to get it under control. It means that maybe you need to start thinking about doing things you'd really rather not do. Like start your kid on Clozapine.

We went back to Dr. Goodman. He listened. He read. He announced that we were going to start on Invega. *Huh? What's Invega?* I almost fell out of my chair.

Dr. Goodman had been telling us for months that Patricia needed to be on Clozapine. He had sent us to see his associate. He had sent us to Boston. After the advice we'd gotten that Clozapine was safe and effective for addressing Patricia's symptoms, how could this guy tell us we were starting Invega? It made no sense.

Invega is a new kind of Risperdal in a high-tech, time-release capsule. Where Risperdal's effective component is manufactured by the patient's liver, with Invega, they do it for you in the laboratory. Now they had a drug they could use on treatment-refractory individuals if some of the previous medication trials took out the liver. Remember all those blood test? They'd been watching the liver. So far, Patricia's was still OK.

Risperdal was one of the medications Dr. Washburn had recommended. It was also the medicine Dr. Barnes said wouldn't work. Incredibly, within a week of starting the Invega, the voices started to go away. They got quieter and quieter. Sometimes, they were gone completely. Patricia noticed. These characters had been with her since the third grade. They were there to keep her company.

She handed me this poem:

> I'll be lonely when they change
> They'll take my friends away
> My true friends who are always there
> Here, there, or anywhere

They help me get to sleep
Keep me company when I wake
Truer friends than these
You just cannot make

I don't need a phone
When they come to call
Don't need a doorbell
Nothing at all

Truer friends than these
You just cannot make
No tokens of your friendship
No brownies to bake

What differs these from "real" friends
Is that they're always there
On a train, on a bus,
Nearly everywhere

Truer friends than these
You just cannot make
When it comes to keeping company
Everyone else is in their wake

And although they're often violent
And I know that that is bad
I'd rather them than nothing
Without them I am sad

And although they're only voices
They're very real to me
And if I had MY way
We'd all just let them be.

I wasn't sure whether I should be rooting for the characters. Or the medication. The medication won. For a while.

∞

Notice there is no "N.O.S." at the end of Patricia's new diagnosis. It was time to figure out why. Just like babies come from storks, diagnoses come from a book: the *DSM-IV*. It's the fourth revision of the *Diagnostic and Statistical Manual of Mental Disorders* put out by the American Psychiatric Association. It describes and sets out the criteria for a whole slew of mental disorders you pray that you or your child never gets. To win a particular diagnosis, you need to admit to a certain number of symptoms in a larger group of possibilities and admit to them persisting for a specific length of time. Maybe one or two of the possibilities must be present. Or maybe some other symptoms or events can't be present.

For example, if I were trying to diagnose "Happiness," I'd require that either a contented affect be present or a big smile plus at least three of these other possibilities: giddiness, joy, ecstasy, cheerfulness, or good humor. These symptoms would need to be present for at least three weeks. The Happiness couldn't be brought on by smoking pot or winning the lottery. And you couldn't be suffering from the more serious Smiley Clown Disorder.

"N.O.S." means "Not Otherwise Specified." They just add it to the end of the diagnosis if all the criteria aren't met. Maybe you've only been happy for a week. Or maybe only joy and good humor are present, but the others aren't. Simply, it means you don't meet the criteria. You don't have it. We'd been into this for nearly a year and so far, my kid has had depressive disorder, but not; bipolar disorder, but not; anxiety disorder, but not; and mood disorder, but not.

"Rule Out" means "maybe." You might have it. Whereas N.O.S. means they have enough information to know you don't meet the criteria, Rule Out means they aren't sure yet. It's like a signal to the next doctor to think about it.

It didn't take me long to figure out why they invented N.O.S.: Treatment. If there is a diagnosis, you can treat. And if there is a diagnosis, you can get services. Without one, you can't get either. To insurance companies and the Department of Mental Health, it's as if N.O.S. is written in invisible ink. They don't care. They can treat. The problem is they can only treat you for what they've already decided you don't have.

How can you get better if they are treating you for something you don't have?

Patricia wasn't getting better. They'd been treating her for depression, anxiety, and bipolar disorders. Maybe we'd have better luck going after something they actually thought she had.

A friend recommended meditation. *Medication? She's already on that.* Not "medication." "Meditation." There is a Buddhist retreat nearby. Maybe she should go there. Turns out they didn't have a program for suicidal 15-year-olds.

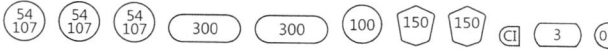

$$- \text{⊲} - \boxed{100} \boxed{100} \boxed{100} + \boxed{3} \boxed{3} - \boxed{100} \boxed{100}$$
$$- \boxed{100} \boxed{100} + \text{⊲} + \boxed{100} - \boxed{100} + \boxed{434} - \boxed{433}$$

Dialectical Behavioral Therapy

Dr. Barnes's report recommended DBT, Dialectical Behavior Therapy. We'd been trying to make this happen ever since the Department of Mental Health offered us a course in it as part of their flexible services menu. DBT was developed by Marsha Linehan, the author of those pages from the *Skills Training Manual for Treating Borderline Personality Disorder* we didn't understand during Patricia's first hospitalization. DBT is a whole range of taught skills, originally intended to keep suicidal young women alive. It has since been adapted for suicidal adolescents.

The goal of DBT is to get through this moment without making things worse. And to do it over and over again. The cool thing is that as long as you can keep doing it, you will never die by suicide. Interesting concept. And something we needed.

Our version of DBT operated as a parent group running concurrently with a teen group. The kids got together once a week for 12 weeks and learned about DBT while their parents met and studied the same things down the hall. There were handouts. There was reading. There was homework. The success of the program is determined largely by how invested the student is in the handouts, the reading, and the homework. Which isn't necessarily easy for a suicidal adolescent. Or their parents. Normally, DBT involves a component with weekly sessions with a DBT-trained individual therapist. Ours didn't work that way. Patricia just had Deb. She was willing to play along.

The first premise of DBT is the unconditional acceptance everyone is trying their hardest and doing their best. As I sat watching the other parents, week after week, only making it to a meeting now and then, and mostly never doing their homework, I knew this acceptance business wasn't going to work for me. I didn't believe for a second these people were trying. They weren't getting anything out of this. I hoped I was.

What we were trying to learn was bizarre. It's a bit of a hodgepodge of Buddhist mindfulness, reality testing, emotion regulation, distress tolerance, and acceptance. We'd start every meeting with a mindfulness exercise. We'd breathe. We'd count our breaths. We'd eat one raisin—in five minutes. We'd walk slowly through the grass, contemplating our steps. We'd be at one with something. Anything. It reminded me of the Lamaze class Kate and I took before Patricia was born.

In DBT, we learned the What Skills. We Observed. We used our Mindfulness Skills to slow down enough to experience what was going on around us. We Described. We learned to see and label what we were Observing. We Participated. Once we were able to Describe what was going on around us, we took the time to fully Participate in it all. Sounds kind of hokey, but it's actually pretty cool.

We learned the How Skills. We tried to be Non-Judgmental; stick to the facts without editorializing about whether it is stupid or not. Our homework for this lesson was to be Mindful of our Thoughts for a day; to recognize when we were jumping to Negative Conclusions about the actions of people around us. I managed to come up with four. Patricia came home from school with a sheet of paper nearly filled with tally marks. They were organized by class: math had 77, physics 90, freshman seminar 88, English 85, Latin 112, and history had 128 tick marks. She said she decided not to keep track during lunch because she was convinced she would run out of paper. I never imagined her classmates annoyed her that much.

We tried to be One-Minded. With the attention span of a gnat, this was a tough one for me. But it's amazing how much more productive I can be if I'm only doing one thing at a time, not 20, particularly when 18 have no practical purpose. We tried to be Effective. Finding what works, and then doing it. Rather than focusing on all the ways we already know don't work.

We learned Interpersonal Effectiveness Skills. Every week we studied another acronym, one of those things where the first letter of each line spells out some secret code word. The first was DEAR MAN, a skill used to help you get what you want. We (D)escribed the problem. We (E)xpressed why it was an issue and what we thought about it. We (A)sserted clearly what we wanted. We (R)einforced our assertion with supporting statements. We stayed (M)indful of our goal and were unwilling to be distracted. We (A)ppeared Confident, even when we weren't. And we (N)egotiated, when appropriate to do so.

We learned GIVE, a skill used in conversations to maintain civil relationships. We tried to be (G)entle. No verbal or physical attacks. Watch the sarcasm. We tried to Act (I)nterested. Apparently, you need to listen to what the other person is saying in order to have a real conversation. *Maybe that's my problem.* Eye contact. *Oh no.* Everybody else tried to (V)alidate. Show sympathy. Understand the other person's point of view. Acknowledge their feelings. I was terrible at this. When I surreptitiously tried this at home on Beth, she turned around, looked me in the eye, and said, "Dad, cut it out." Apparently, I had never validated anything Beth had ever said or done. She noticed when I tried. And she knew it was fake. We tried to use an (E)asy Manner. Smile. Calm and comfortable. Not very easy for someone who doesn't even know how to validate.

We learned FAST, another skill designed to help maintain your self-respect. We were (F)air to everyone. We didn't Over (A)pologize. We (S)tuck to our values. And we were (T)ruthful.

After a while, they all started to blur together. Trying to incorporate these things into real life was difficult. Without a crib sheet, I certainly couldn't keep track of all the steps. Beth saw right through me in one second. Imagine if I had stopped to get out my notes. Or had them written on the back of my hand.

But of course we weren't done. We moved on to the Emotion Regulation Skills. But we were running out of time. So we skipped the PLEASE skills and went right on to Opposite Action, which I never really understood, Problem Solving, and Letting Go. It turns out that if you are justified in your anger at something or someone, and you actually do something about it, the sense of relief is real. And if you can't bring yourself to actually do something, if you just notice your anger and label it, you can get nearly the same relief by just letting it go. It's incompatible with holding a grudge, but if you can actually bring yourself to move on, the effect is satisfying.

DBT's Distress Tolerance Skills were most useful for Patricia. With how she was feeling, she was in distress nearly every second of every waking moment. She wanted to be dead. She wanted to cut. The medications weren't helping. Therapy hadn't solved it. The choice was either to kill herself or figure out how to cope with her feeling for just this moment. Patricia worked very hard finding ways to tolerate her circumstances. Most of the time, she found a way to do it without cutting.

The ACCEPTS Skills kept Patricia alive. She searched for (A)ctivities she enjoyed. She (C)ontributed by helping others in the community. She made (C)omparisons between herself and others. She actually was able to identify people who were doing worse than she was. She sought out Other (E)motions. Good feelings. To try to overwhelm the bad ones. To (P)ush Away what was going on with her and doing something else for a while. To concentrate on Other (T)houghts. And distract with Other Intense (S)ensations.

Over the next couple of years, I took the DBT course three times. Patricia took it again with Kate. Beth took it once with me as we tried to include her in what was going on with her sister. Beth was particularly fond of DEAR MAN. She used it for the longest time trying to convince her parents to buy her a cell phone. Apparently she was paying attention to (M)indfulness, because she was relentless in her pursuit of that phone. She never gave up. I admired her determination. It never changed my mind about when she needed one, but I was impressed with her ability to remain focused on the prize.

I discovered a set of skills that work for me. I should use them more often. The mindfulness breathing exercises are my ticket to real relaxation. Focusing on the breath in and on the breath out. Counting them. Returning focus every time my mind wanders, which is often. Trying to stay in the moment. If you can do it without giggling about how stupid it is, it really works. But being non-judgmental is part of DBT. *I'm not very good at that.*

For me, the "S" part of ACCEPTS works pretty well, too. Other Intense (S)ensations. A very hot shower or really loud music is a great way to dissipate the building anger associated with what's going on around me. Certain kinds of rap or dance music, in the car, cranked until just before my ears start bleeding, can calm me and get me out of whatever rut my family has careened us into.

And DBT taught me a new way to eat junk food at the movies. I can now eat one Peanut M&M in the time most people eat a whole bag (yes, the big movie-theatre-sized bag). The problem is that if I share them with my movie-going mate, I only get one. Not very satisfying.

Finally, DEAR MAN has helped me have the strength to ask for and even demand the help we have needed to keep Patricia safe.

DBT added a whole array of skills to Patricia's safety plan. Many of them kept her closer to home or around people. Taking a shower. Going to a movie. Clutching a frozen orange is a great distraction. It's cold to the touch. The surface gets a little slimy as you handle it as it warms up. The smell permeates.

Mostly, DBT has kept Patricia alive. Unfortunately, it didn't actually solve anything. But it gave her the strength to get through some very unpleasant moments.

∞

And Patricia was having lots of unpleasant moments.

We talked with DMH regularly. Keeping them up to speed on how badly things were going. They tried very hard to be helpful. They suggested "respite." It's another one of the flexible services they offered. "Respite" means "break." Or "interlude." Sometimes it's designed to give the kid a break. Sometimes it's designed to give the parents one. In our case, the offer was for Patricia to spend some Friday and Saturday nights at Greendale Youth Services, a nearby residential and day treatment program.

Greendale has a number of different kinds of "Beds." Some are "IRTP Beds," long-term beds for kids in a DMH sponsored Intensive Residential Treatment Program. Others are "Step-down Beds," shorter-term ones for kids transitioning from an inpatient hospital stay to home. A couple are DMH "Respite Beds."

Think about the first day your parents dropped you off at preschool. You were pretty young back then. Not a whole lot of language skills. Crying was still the major means of communicating that this is not a place you want to be. "Please don't leave me here." "I choose to stay with you rather than be left here with these piranhas." Imagine, if on that day, you had another 10 years of language arts education. Imagine you'd gotten straight A's for all those years. Imagine you'd just covered the DEAR MAN skills in your DBT class. And you were getting pretty good at the (M)indfulness letter. Now imagine what might happen when your parents tried to drop you off at that first day of preschool.

Patricia wasn't too keen on the idea of respite. Kate and I thought it was a good idea. Something to try. Patricia wasn't buying it. "I don't want to go to respite." *You might like it.* "I don't want to go to respite." *Who knows, you might have fun.* We didn't quite say she was going anyway, but she went anyway.

We got in the car and drove to Greendale. "I don't want to go to respite." We pulled into the parking lot. "I don't want to go to respite." We went inside. "Please take me home." It felt just like we were leaving her at preschool for the first time.

Kate and I drove home.

The phone was ringing when we walked in the door. Guess what? It was Patricia. "Please come get me." "I don't want to be here." This went on, every two hours, for the next day and a half — even at two and four a.m. She was relentless. It got old pretty fast. There was a staff person with her when she made these calls. Every once in a while, I asked to speak with him. We talked about how this was fairly typical behavior for some of their kids. About how Kate and I needed to decide if we were going to come get the child. About how the staff wasn't allowed to make any recommendations. It was up to the family. About how, yes, this was a difficult decision. And thankfully, about how we wouldn't be labeled bad parents if we continued to say no and left her there.

The calls continued the next day. "I don't want to be here." "Please come get me." "Next time, just book me a room in Hell. It would be better than this." *Be strong. Just say no.*

At some point, she gave up. But by then it was nearly time to bring her home. When I walked in the door at Greendale, I think she might have scowled at me. For the first time in her life.

She never went back to respite.

School was finishing up for the year. One afternoon I was feeling a little cocky. I decided to see if Patricia could make it through the day without being coddled. Kate was back to work some days. I decided not to be home when Patricia got out of school. Big mistake. "Of all the days to not be home for me after school and not let me know, today was not the day." *Busted.*

The story was that Patricia's friends hated her. This had been going on for a couple of days. She tried to find out why. They wouldn't tell her. She was devastated. Somehow, if I had been home, it would have been better. But I wasn't. The next day, Patricia sucked it up and went back to school. And asked again. And they told her why they hated her. Apparently, it wasn't such a big deal. Nothing she could fix. Nothing important. Patricia came home feeling great. She was pleased to have friends she could have normal spats with. I was there to greet her when she got home.

That day. And many more to come.

Patricia started having weird dreams. We made a list:

Patricia's Dreams

- ☐ *Vanilla flavored orange juice. They came up with the recipe at school.*
- ☐ *Glade PlugIns argument with dad. Patricia for. Dad against.*
- ☐ *Someone tried to make me eat veal.*
- ☐ *Mom had another stroke. She didn't survive.*

The characters were still gone. It had been more than a week since she started on Invega. Patricia was lonely. Still. She had trouble getting to sleep: "They aren't there to keep me company." She didn't want to walk the dog. Again, no one to keep her company. She thought about cutting. But didn't. "That's stupid. Don't do that." She thought about Brian. And her belt. And the game "tingle."

The characters came back after nine days. Dr. Goodman added some more medication and they were gone again. Lonely. Anxious. Claustrophobic. Carbohydrate cravings. "Is celery OK?" Yes.

Patricia started tapping her knee. Or maybe her knee starting tapping itself.

"I can't get to sleep."

Patricia started reading again. She would read more than 2,000 pages over the next few weeks. Significantly more than she had read in the entire last year. Nearly as much as she used to read. Maybe she'd be able to function in school when it started in the fall. Dr. Goodman tweaked the meds again.

She slept. Magnificently. And woke refreshed and alert.

However, Patricia started wetting the bed. That hadn't happened since she was three.

She was exhausted during the day. We moved her bedtime earlier. And her wakeup time later. We could do this because it was now summer; this wasn't going to work for school.

We had a few good days.

"I wish I was dead." No reason. No slow decline. Just from fine to, "I wish I was dead." I found comfort that it wasn't, "I want to be dead." By now, I knew the difference.

Deb was getting harder to reach. It seemed the voice mailbox was always full. We really needed some thoughtful advice.

∞

Reader, it's time to stop again for a moment and regroup. We're on page 116. It's summer. We've survived just one year of high school. As long as you didn't skip Patricia's introduction at the beginning of the book, you already know she makes it through another three. But it will take a while to get there. I found some stuff on the Internet to paint on the ends of my oak-tree lumber to protect it from cracking while it spent a couple of years drying out. I wish I had something to protect Patricia as she tried to grow up. Our stories are long and complicated. We are going to give them the time they need. Maybe you should go to bed now. We won't be able to finish this tonight.

(54/107) (54/107) (54/107) (150) (150) (C) (9) (433) (0)

$$+ \; + \; - \; + \; +/- \; - \; \boxed{433} \; + \; \boxed{100}$$

$$- \boxed{\tfrac{54}{107}} - \boxed{100} - \; + \; \boxed{4359} - \boxed{\tfrac{54}{107}} - \; + \; \boxed{4359} \; \boxed{4359} \; \boxed{4359}$$

$$- \boxed{\tfrac{54}{107}} - \boxed{C110} \; -/+ \; + \; \boxed{7772} \; + \; \boxed{7772}$$

Starting Sophomore Year

School started. Sophomore year.

It was clear that Patricia was heading back to the hospital. All I could do was watch it play out and do my best to make sure it happened in a safe and controlled way. I started making more detailed notes. I wanted to get the words just right. We had a treatment plan. It was in writing. It was progressing just like Dr. Barnes had said it would: "Risperdal won't work. Clozapine will." We were going the route that wouldn't work. And wasn't.

Clozapine was on deck.

Everything got dark. Patricia turned up the lights. "Now everything has a purple tinge.

"I'm safe. But I'm preoccupied with death and suicide.

"I keep thinking about antifreeze and overdosing again.

"I want to go to bed so I don't have to think about it."

I asked her if she wanted to go to EMH. "It's probably a good idea, but I told you I won't go to the hospital again." That's right. She did say that. I was there. But I didn't think she was serious. And that was before I was writing everything down.

"I'm safe.

"I want to cut; but I won't."

I asked her if the characters were back. "I'm not sure. Maybe." "They might be when I'm asleep, but that doesn't count."

She calculated her BMI for health class. *Uh-oh.*

"I wish I hadn't read Brian's story. I'm thinking about how to hang myself." "I can't stop thinking about it." "I wish I was in the hospital so they can put me on a new antidepressant and I won't do anything during the change."

I called Deb and left a message. She called me back. I think that all the colorful material I included in my message is what precipitated the callback. We talked for a while. I told her how impressed I was at how well Patricia was reporting her feelings to me. I told her I was amazed at how Patricia still managed to be in school nearly every day with everything going on inside her. I told her I was in awe at how long Patricia was managing to hang on without going to the hospital. Deb asked me if I thought it was fair to let Patricia go through what she was going through when the hospital just might be the place that could actually make her feel better. The goal isn't to keep her out of the hospital. The goal is for her to be better. *Dope. She was right.*

I started making copies of Dr. Barnes's report. I did my best to update Patricia's clinical history. I started concocting a medication log to memorialize all her medication changes.

"I just want to get it over and kill myself.

"I could take a rope and make a slipknot.

"I don't want to go to sleep. When you sleep, your creative mind works. I don't want to get any ideas."

To school. To another doctor—a geneticist. To talk about how Patricia's body metabolizes all the medications she is taking. Can it still be a good appointment even if we didn't understand anything? At this point, I'll take any positive news. Back to school. Home. To Beth's soccer practice. Home. To bed.

Not the sleep kind of bed. The under the covers kind.

Patricia sat in bed, under the covers, and thought about what to do next.

"I'm not leaving here until I know what I'm going to do."

Shower? "No, I will cut."

What if you move the razor before you take your shower? "No. I can't get close enough to the razor to move it. I'm staying here."

Laundry? "No. I'll drink the bleach."

Maybe you should go to another room. "There might be a string or rope in there."

Kate walked by her room, noticed her there in bed, and asked how she was doing?

"Fine."

Do your Latin homework.

"OK."

Patricia did her Latin homework. Recovered remarkably. And went to bed content.

The next morning she was back to feeling awful. Off to school.

Near noon, she went to see Mrs. Harris in the guidance office. They talked about how Patricia was doing. "Badly." Patricia decided to implement her Safety Plan.

This was incredible! There was a Safety Plan. And Patricia decided it was time to put it into action.

They made a list of things to talk about with Deb later that day. And then Patricia went back to class. She and Mrs. Harris decided Patricia would finish the day at school. She was safe there. And she wanted to go to the second meeting of the Latin Club that was getting together after school. She would be safe there too. Mrs. Harris called me up and told me the plan: Please be there to pick Patricia up at school after Latin Club.

I was there to pick her up after Latin Club.

"I have given up hope."

We went to see Deb for a few minutes on our way to EMH.

I called Dr. Goodman and left a message. He called me back and said that Invega had been given a fair trial. Patricia needs to be on Clozapine. And she needs to be inpatient—not emergency respite.

EMH was understanding. They knew Patricia by now. We still waited hours to see someone, but when we did, they had already read everything from the last three times she'd been there. I gave them copies of Patricia's medication history, the letter from Dr. Barnes, an updated clinical history, and Dr. Goodman's recommendations for inpatient hospitalization and Clozapine.

Twelve hours later, she was back at Patriot Medical. I met the ambulance there. We'd already packed some clothes, some books, and the stuffed moose, so Patricia had everything she needed. As I was getting ready to leave, I confirmed that all the paperwork and notes I'd given to the doctor at EMH had traveled with Patricia to Patriot Medical.

But by now, you must know they hadn't. Nope. Lost.

I knew this was going to happen. I had an extra copy. I left it all with the intake nurse, went home and slept. The next day, I found my place at the end of Patricia's bed.

Usually, the act of landing in the hospital had some restorative effect on Patricia. She'd be a little better when I came to visit for the first time. But not this time. Patricia said she had "self-injurious hopes." *Huh?* She translated for me: It means she wishes to harm herself and will be pleased if she is able to accomplish her goal. That's what she said. I had hoped it wasn't what she meant. Unfortunately, it was.

I alerted the staff to her mood. Maybe I'd win another Anxious Father Award.

As I was getting ready to leave for the day, I stopped at the desk and spoke with the head nurse. I asked about Patricia's medications. I wanted to know if anyone had read all the paperwork that came in with Patricia and if they had started her on Clozapine. The nurse looked in her chart. There was a handwritten medication list, but nothing else. No paperwork. No reports from Dr. Barnes. The nurse said Patricia been given all the medications on the list, except for Invega. She had never heard of that. So she didn't give her any.

This is when the normal person would start shouting. Start breaking windows and kidnapping the kid to get her away from there and to somewhere safe. I decided to bite my tongue and do this methodically. I explained to the nurse that Invega is one of those antipsychotics you can't just stop taking without carefully tapering it? She checked. *Yup.*

Except.

Except they don't have any and can't get any for a day or two. The nurse asked me if I had some. *Sure. At home.* "Could you go get it?" *OK.* I got in the car and drove home to get some Invega and another copy of all the paperwork.

I was getting worried. It was getting to be late on Friday. Patricia had been working her way into the hospital for more than 24 hours. They weren't exuding a lot of confidence in their ability to help her. I started making calls. By now, I had enough phone numbers to call that some people actually answered their phone. The consensus was I should confirm that Patriot Medical was familiar with Invega and Clozapine. If not, get her into someplace that is. But do it carefully, because with your insurance, Patriot Medical is going to have to agree with a decision to move her because they are going to have to pay—and they will want to keep her where she is unless you can convince them she won't be safe.

So far, I was doing pretty well: I had a kid whose goal was to hurt herself and a head nurse who had never heard of Invega. This was going to be easy.

When I got back to the hospital, most of the regular staff was gone. The weekend aides and babysitters had taken over. My question would need to wait until Monday.

On Saturday morning, I learned that the hospital psychiatrist had changed Patricia's medications the previous night before going home for the weekend. *Isn't the treatment team supposed to talk with the parents before they do that?*

I might have forgiven them if they had started her on Clozapine. But they hadn't.

Patricia had a rough weekend. Everything was dark again. Like dusk. She asked me to buy her a stress ball—a heavy-duty two-inch balloon filled with sand. She'd been clutching ice cubes to try to overcome her "self-injurious thoughts." She wanted to cut. But didn't have anything to cut with. She asked the hospital staff if she could draw cuts on her arm with a red pen. They said, "No." They did give her a couple of elastic bands to put on her wrist and snap. That actually helped. Lots.

Some of the staff started talking with Patricia as if she would be going off to a "Program." Nobody told her what a "Program" was. Patricia went to pieces.

The characters were back. She had missed them.

Her wrist was numb from snapping the elastics.

She was having nightmares about a "Program."

She was miserable.

She was tippy.

She was slightly too happy.

All at the same time.

Sitting at the end of her bed, Patricia told me she wasn't so sure about this Clozapine idea. She worried about the kids at school thinking she was a heroin addict because of all the track marks on her arms from the weekly blood draws. I chose to ignore this comment.

Monday came around. It took them until 5:00 p.m. to find the letters from Dr. Barnes, Patricia's history, and the medication list. They were in the social worker's inbox. No one had looked at them. Patricia had been in the hospital nearly four days. Wasn't that the total length of an average stay? And they hadn't even read the paperwork on the patient? *This was stupid.*

I asked the social worker to find out if the hospital knew anything about Invega and Clozapine. She went off to check. She came back later and told me that the parent of one of the current Children's Psychiatric Unit patients was taking Invega. But they knew nothing about it. She told me that the hospital does not prescribe Clozapine. This was getting stupider. Why did it matter that the parent of one of the patients was on Invega? And why was Patricia sent to a hospital that doesn't prescribe Clozapine if she needs to be on Clozapine?

Clearly, this was the wrong place for Patricia. She needed to be somewhere else. I started making calls. I called Leslie Steiner, my contact at Mystic Valley Healthcare. She said Cambridge Hospital and McLean know how to prescribe Clozapine for adolescents. Step two was to figure out how to get her out of Patriot Medical and into somewhere else. I called one of my parent support partners. She told me about something called the "Peace of Mind Clause." I'm not sure if it actually exists, but the parent partner told me that when all else fails, just invoke it. Tell the hospital your child is unsafe there. Tell them your kid is moving. And then act like it is going to happen. I called my insurance company and asked to talk with a supervisor again. She listened with interest to my story. She seemed very understanding. She said to talk with Patriot Medical. Tell them everything that I had just told her. Ask them what they are going to do about it. Ultimately, they are responsible for treating her there or finding someplace that can.

I decided to gather some more evidence before I talked with Patriot Medical. Besides, everyone was too busy to talk with me anyway.

Patricia was worse. She wanted to cut. The hospital staff said no. She saw nothing wrong with it. They said cutting is a coping skill that doesn't work. Choose another one. Except suicide. They said she should have some coping skills to use for when she wants to cut. "What about my safety plan? Isn't that what it's for?" They told her she should take a DBT class. She burst into tears. She had already taken that. It wasn't working.

Patricia starting reporting suicidal thoughts to the staff.

The next day Patricia told me, "If you take me home, I will break away, run upstairs, and cut. No matter what." Going home wasn't on the list of possibilities, so for once, I didn't worry.

Patricia wasn't getting better. She'd been in the hospital for nearly a week. She continued to get worse. It was getting to the point where we should have scheduled a discharge meeting to talk about taking her home. But we still hadn't scheduled the intake meeting to talk about what they were going to do for Patricia while she was there. I asked if I could speak with the hospital psychiatrist. I had enough ammunition to make a case for moving Patricia. She agreed to meet later that day.

We met.

I told her I was disappointed Patricia had been here for nearly a week and I didn't think anyone had read any of the paperwork that came along with her. We had a treatment plan. It needed implementing. Their hospital didn't do Clozapine. Nothing had been done. Patricia was getting worse.

The doctor told me she had read the material and supported the plan to start Patricia on Clozapine. Patricia was a worthy candidate. She handed me some photocopied information about Clozapine, asked that I read it, share it with Patricia, and said it would start tomorrow after the blood test results were in. And by the way, "I need Patricia's Social Security number so I can register her with the Clozapine National Registry."

Our meeting did not go as I had planned.

∞

This is the point in our story where, normally, we'd take a bit of a break. We'd go off on a tangent and ruminate about something that has nothing to do with anything. Then I'd try to twist it around and make a point about just how unbelievable what just happened really is. About how I'm at a loss for words. Unfortunately, there is no story in my half century of collected experiences to properly demonstrate how I didn't have any idea how to react to the hospital's announcement that Patricia was starting on Clozapine. I was speechless. If I could, do I say, "Thank you," and get over it? Do I still get her out of there? Does this change everything? Is she really in the right place after all?

I was at a loss for words.

But if I leave this detour out, then you'll never know.

So instead, I'm going to tell you the story of our family trip back to "Newfoundland." Maybe it does apply.

Kate and I had been to Newfoundland just before Patricia was born. It was time to go back. The children were old enough to appreciate the incredible scenery. They were also six and nine. Which means they were old enough to hate each other's guts. Putting them in the car together was like throwing gasoline on an already raging wildfire.

They squabbled.

To put it mildly.

So before I agreed to this trip, I did the math. Just how long would we be stuck in the car together? I added it all up. If you count the ferries, it's about 2,000 miles, round-trip, from Massachusetts to Newfoundland. Wow. I did some more math. If we were willing to drive 2,000 miles, we could make it to Denver and back. So why didn't we just drive to Denver instead? I did some more research. The reason you don't drive from Massachusetts to Denver and back is simple: It's boring. Nothing to see except some cornfields. Plenty of opportunity to concentrate on squabbling.

So instead of driving to Newfoundland—or Denver, we flew to Denver, took a daylight train ride through the Rockies to Salt Lake City, rented a car, and drove back to Denver—by a circuitous route. The kids floated in the Great Salt Lake, we drove the Going-to-the-Sun Road through Glacier National Park, we went to Yellowstone, the Grand Tetons, and drove through 2,000 miles of purple majesty. During this time, the children didn't fight once. They sat in the back seat. Breathless. Mesmerized. Every time we went around another corner and the view changed, they emitted a guttural "Ooh," or "Aah." For 2,000 miles.

They were at a loss for words.

There is more than one way to become speechless.

I was at a loss for words.

I like the purple majesty way of getting my breath taken away rather than the one from talking with the psychiatrist at the mental hospital.

∞

Patricia started on Clozapine.

I was there for the first dose. The nurse came in, handed Patricia a pill and a glass of water. Patricia swallowed the pill. The nurse said it was Clozapine. OK. Patricia and I looked at each other. Within a few seconds, I found an excuse to leave her room for a moment. I found the head nurse and asked her about the Clozapine pill Patricia had just been given. I told her that the paperwork the doctor gave us the day before, in the dispensing instructions, said to let the pill dissolve on your tongue, without water, without chewing, and without swallowing. If so, why did the nurse have her swallow this new pill? "I'll check." A few minutes later, she came back and told me they had given Patricia a different kind of pill. The kind you swallow. I was pretty sure Patricia had read the paperwork, knew she wasn't supposed to swallow it, and was now completely freaking out in her room. I asked the nurse to go talk with Patricia about her new medicine. She agreed. When she came back a minute later, she told me Patricia was relieved to hear that it was a different kind of Clozapine. She had been freaking out in her room.

They started to slowly taper some of Patricia's other medications. When the nurse said that she had cut the Invega capsules in half to begin reducing the dose, I almost fell off the end of Patricia's bed. Once again, I went into the other room and asked the head nurse if she had read the Invega directions. The ones that caution against cutting the capsules. The high-tech coating meters the dose throughout the day. If it's damaged, you get the whole thing at once.

It took a number of days to get Patricia safely switched to Clozapine. But it only took a couple of days for her to start feeling better. By day 10 of Patricia's hospital stay, Patricia seemed to be responding well.

"I think the characters are responsible for my depression. I think I will feel better if they are gone." Amazing. It was the first thing she'd said that made any sense in nearly a month.

"I'm feeling better.

"I don't want to kill myself today.

"I'm safe. I promise I'll wait until my 18th birthday to kill myself."

A couple of days later, she was feeling pretty good. Laughing. She had just been kicked out of group. They were playing Twenty Questions. Apparently she was getting all the answers right. She was monopolizing the group. So they kicked her out to give the other kids a chance. They promised to let her back in for the next game. It made her feel great. Her competitive edge resurfaced.

But there were side-effects. Just like usual. But they weren't any worse than anything else she'd been through. Headaches. Feeling a little queasy now and then. A little bit distant. The Clozapine was sedating. She was getting restful and restorative sleep. But she was sleeping during the day, too. They moved her morning Clozapine to before bedtime.

The anxiety was still there. But it seemed to be developing a pattern. It wasn't every second of every day. Now it was related to what was going on around her. She was fine one day. But the next day, when one of the 12-year-old girls on the ward started shouting and running and trying to cut, Patricia asked for her anxiety PRN to help calm down. That and snapping the elastic bands on her wrists did the trick. The next day, when one of the boys on the ward had his hissy-fit, Patricia's anxiety wasn't that bad. The characters returned long enough to keep her company while he ranted and raved.

The characters were on their way out, but they were leaving a bloody swath as they went. "The characters have started killing off my friends." *Who?* "Nathan. So far." *How?* "I don't want to talk about it." A few days later, all her friends were dead. Killed. One at a time. By those same characters who had been telling her stories inside her head for years. Her friends were gone. The unfriendly characters wouldn't go away. It didn't seem fair.

∞

I don't want you to think I didn't notice Patricia said she would wait until her 18th birthday to kill herself. I heard it. She said it during a time of lucid dialogue. She also said she was safe. Her demeanor changed. She had made an important decision.

Her 18th birthday was two and a half years away. That's a long time. DBT is designed to keep you safe in the moment—just for this one second. If you string a whole bunch of those seconds together, before you know it, you have a long and bearable (or miserable) life. If Patricia was serious, and I believed she was, she had just told me she would be safe for more than 75 million seconds. Seventy-five million DBT moments. *Wow.*

I took great comfort in this statement. It took me a long time to begin thinking about how I might feel after those 75 million moments were nearly gone. Because I was too busy appreciating today's.

∞

The hospital announced they had started the process to file an "IRTP" application on Patricia. "IRTP" stands for "Intensive Residential Treatment Program." A "Program." *Oh.* Like they have at Greendale Youth Services. *Goody. Something to look forward to.* The IRTP process sets out a course of action for evaluating the kid to see if she meets the criteria for needing a longer-term residential placement. The hospital writes a letter to the Department of Mental Health recommending placement. And then DMH does an independent evaluation. In the meantime, everyone stops talking about going home. The insurance company temporarily loses its voice. They just shut up and pay.

An IRTP application is a little like your driver's license picture: Once you take it, you are stuck with it. And it comes back to haunt you until it has finished serving its purpose. Even if that purpose is to show you who you really are. The fact that Patricia was getting better had no effect on the IRTP process. The fact that they decided to start the IRTP process on the day they actually began treating her with the medicine everyone who was involved in her care knew was next on the list and might have actually helped her not need residential placement in the first place had no effect on anything. (Sorry about the run-on sentence; I was starting to get mad.) Nothing was going to sidetrack the IRTP process.

And the process is slow.

Going home was still off the list.

Patricia was reading again, so she picked up the first book in the *Harry Potter* series and started reading. One book every couple of days.

The school sent her some homework every once in a while. She did everything they asked. She still had plenty of time to read.

DMH arranged for one of their consulting psychiatrists to meet with her. But he couldn't do his thing until the hospital finished their application letter. And the hospital was slow. In the meantime, I sent him a copy of all the paperwork.

On day 20 of Patricia's hospitalization, a Thursday, a big meeting was held. Dr. Chase was there. And the social worker. The hospital psychiatrist popped in. She had spoken with Dr. Goodman before the meeting. And even though he hadn't received the IRTP application from the hospital, the DMH psychiatrist attended. Although he wasn't officially on the case, he took charge of the meeting. He talked about Patricia's auditory hallucinations. He felt that the frequency and timing of them were important. He asked the social worker to get together with Patricia and set up a daily log to track them so that he would have a history when he met with Patricia the next week. She agreed.

By the next day, the hospital had finally finished the IRTP application and sent it off to DMH. I was in the hallway talking with the hospital psychiatrist about it. As she glanced at the report, she commented to me that she was surprised to see that it said that the auditory hallucinations were present three times each day. *Of course they were. That's what we spent most of yesterday's meeting talking about.* But wait. She wasn't there for the whole meeting. She just popped in now and then.

I probed. I wanted to find out what the psychiatrist really knew about what was going on. Ultimately, I decided that as of today, day 21 of Patricia's hospitalization, she still hadn't read Dr. Barnes's report or the recent family history. I spent a couple of seconds trying to convince myself it didn't matter; she could treat Patricia even if she didn't have that information. But I couldn't believe what I was hearing. And I couldn't believe that what I was hearing could be justified under any circumstances.

Friday came to an end. Everyone went home for the weekend. Patricia finished another *Harry Potter* book. And started another. I went back to my station at the end of Patricia's bed. And fumed. And fumed.

I'm not very good at small talk. Indubitably, our conversations end up with me asking Patricia how she's feeling. Me gathering facts. I asked how her log was going for the DMH psychiatrist. "What log?" *Didn't the social worker talk to you about starting one?* "When?" *Yesterday, after the meeting.* "No."

∞

This is supposed to be a story about Patricia. About what's going on in her life. About the therapeutic services she was getting in the hospital. About how what she was learning from the caring and dedicated staff would serve her as she returned to the community. Instead, it seems to be a story about Patricia re-reading the *Harry Potter* books and doing homework every once in a while. If I were the insurance company, I'd be annoyed.

I tried to have a conversation with the social worker about this. Incredibly, she agreed with me. Yup. Patricia really isn't getting anything out of this. But instead of stepping up to the plate and fixing it, she told me that their program was no longer appropriate for Patricia. It repeats. Remember *Mental Health, the Musical*? There is only six days of material. Patricia had been through it nearly four times during this hospital stay. She wasn't going to get anything more out of it.

Within a couple of days, the hospital heard from the Department of Mental Health. Their psychiatrist had concluded Patricia was not a danger to herself or to others, and therefore, she was not an appropriate candidate for an IRTP placement. A report would follow shortly.

I learned of this in the social worker's office. She had called me in there to say Patricia was ready to go home.

Hold it a second. Something wasn't right. *The same kid they had filed an IRTP application on was ready to go home?* "Yes" *When?* "Today." *Why?* "DMH says she doesn't meet the criteria for placement in a long-term residential program." *OK. Where should she go?* "We haven't seen his report, yet." *Where do you recommend?* "Home." I asked them to write a letter with their recommendations.

Hospitals are slow. It took them another couple of weeks to finish their paperwork. Patricia stayed right where she was. Reading *Harry Potter*. And doing some schoolwork every now and then.

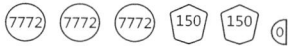

Finding Another School

It was early November. So far this fall, Patricia had been in school for two weeks. She'd been in the hospital for six and a half. She came home with a short list of personal goals:

- ☐ *I need to ease slowly back into school.*
- ☐ *I need to be in a different school: One that understands me.*
- ☐ *I want to be included in the decision-making process.*

She also came home with a new understanding of herself: "I'm a nervous person." Nervous about today. Every today. "Nervous that if I don't do well today, I'll be doomed tomorrow." And nervous about the report she needs to do for school that is due next week.

For the today stuff, she didn't have any options. She was miserable. But she had a strategy for next week's project: Just forget about it until two days before it is due. That way she wouldn't obsess over it for the whole week. Just for the couple of days it would take to get it done. And because Patricia was functioning well enough to actually accomplish things, two days was always long enough to do whatever needed doing.

Patricia's parents came home from the hospital with a veritable goldmine of stuff: Letters. Reports. Forms. Perhaps the most important was a letter from the hospital recommending a placement at a therapeutic day school, whatever that is. We had copies of the original IRTP letter recommending the residential placement, which was now off the table. We had the DMH psychiatrist's report. The only thing surprising in it was that Patricia had admitted to experiencing visual hallucinations. We knew about auditory and olfactory ones, but we hadn't heard about the visual ones. *Uh-oh.* And we had a Physician's Statement for Temporary Home or Hospital Education. This was supposed to get Patricia in-home tutoring until we figured out what to do next. We had the handwritten hospital discharge form—the written one wouldn't be done for months. And we had a copy of an echocardiogram, or ECG report. It's a piece of paper with a bunch of squiggles on it showing Patricia's heart function. The hospital did the test on Patricia as a part of the start of her new medications. The hospital wanted Patricia's primary care physician to interpret it. Apparently, Patricia's heart rate was slightly elevated and maybe some of those squiggles didn't look quite right. And besides, it would take another couple of days for a doctor at Patriot Medical to look at it. They wanted Patricia gone by then.

The school demanded another meeting before Patricia came back to school. Until now, Patricia had been going to school under a 504 Plan. That had given her a couple of accommodations. I knew by now that in order to get a placement in a therapeutic school, Patricia would need a full-blown "IEP," an "Individual Education Plan." To make sure our meeting would include a discussion about the possibility of an IEP and not just revising the 504 Plan, I wrote a letter to the school requesting an IEP meeting. It was just one paragraph long:

> "I would like to request a meeting to discuss the need for an IEP for my daughter, Patricia. She has a 504 Plan. We have concerns that she may need more supports."

I hand delivered a copy to Brenda Harris in the guidance office. I told her another copy would be coming by US Mail, Return Receipt Requested. She said, "Great." She knew that I knew I had the right to request this meeting. And by doing so, the school was required to act within a specified time. By documenting everything in writing, all the proper clocks would start ticking. Mrs. Harris didn't take offense that I was trying to play by the rules.

The school called and said they wanted to do some testing before the meeting. I signed an Evaluation and Consent Form giving them permission to do educational and psychological testing on Patricia. Less than two days after coming home from a six and a half week hospital stay, I dropped Patricia off at the high school so the school psychologist could put her under a microscope. I wondered whether Patricia was in the best frame of mind to be taking all these tests. I wasn't sure if today was the right day to be taking an IQ test. The school psychologist asked me to fill out a 150-question form called the Behavioral Assessment System for Children – Parent Rating Scales about Patricia. I didn't like the questions. I particularly didn't like my answers. Patricia filled out the kid-patient version.

Within a couple of days, we received an invitation to an IEP meeting. Along with it came an attendance sign-up sheet listing everyone who was scheduled to attend. So far. They asked for names of anyone else we might invite. Based on the number of people they were bringing, I think they wanted to know if we needed to move the meeting to the local civic center. It was going to be crowded. Maybe I could talk my sister into coming. Or someone from DMH.

I started hearing horror stories about IEP meetings, particularly those seeking placement in a therapeutic school. Therapeutic schools are expensive. And because our school district doesn't operate any therapeutic schools, this means an "out-of-district placement." Out-of-district therapeutic schools are even more expensive. And the price goes higher still because the school district has to provide door-to-door transportation to the out-of-district school. The school pays for all of this. And they do so either by raising my neighbors' taxes or by cutting programs in the regular schools that are trying their hardest to educate Beth and all my neighbors' children. The consensus was that this IEP meeting would end with a denial for a therapeutic placement. The next step is to sue. Years later, when everyone is exhausted and out of money, if the child is still alive and hasn't aged out of the system, the placement is granted. Now would have been the perfect time to preemptively hire an "educational advocate." Or a lawyer. Once again, I decided to let Patricia's illness speak for itself.

We went off to Dr. Fitzgerald to talk about the ECG. She looked it over and declared that everything was fine. We brought her up to speed on Patricia's recent hospitalization. We talked about the impending IEP meeting. "When is it?" *Next Tuesday.* "Where?" *At the high school.* "I've never been to an IEP meeting before. Tuesday is my day off."

Tuesday came. We all showed up for the IEP meeting. Someone went to get more chairs. Mrs. Harris, the guidance counselor, was our hostess, but she wasn't really in charge—Barton Comstock, the special education specialist, was. We introduced ourselves around the table. Mr. Comstock. Next to him was the special education liaison. Then the guidance counselor, the head of counseling services, the school psychologist, the school nurse, the special education coordinator, the assistant principal, and the program director. Our side of the table had Patricia, mom, dad, my sister, and our case manager from the Department of Mental Health.

We were out-gunned. But we had Patricia on our side—the only one who really mattered.

Except. Dr. Fitzgerald walked in. The pediatrician. Incredible! Someone went to get her a chair.

The school psychologist distributed her report and summarized her findings: Patricia is smart. (I knew that.) She has above-average to superior intelligence. (About the 87th percentile ... gee ... I knew that, too.) She tests better at math than English, yet both are quite high. (Strange ... I thought it was the other way around.)

Based on the Behavior Assessment Patricia completed on herself, the psychologist identified a number of areas of concern: atypicality (acts strangely/hallucinations), social stress (uneasy around others), anxiety (nervousness/irrational fears/worries about making mistakes), depression (sadness/feeling overwhelmed/ lonely), inadequacy (low self-esteem), somatization (headaches/ imagined pain), hyperactivity (rushes through things), and difficulties with interpersonal relationships (trouble making friends) were the big ones. My father-reported behavioral ratings identified similar areas of significant concern, but added withdrawal (shyness/avoidance) and trouble performing activities of daily living. Apparently having difficulty getting up in the morning and wearing the same clothes, day after day, no matter what the weather, is a problem. I always thought that was part of the definition of "adolescent." *Or me.*

The psychologist's report went on to say that high school has been a significant source of stress for Patricia and seems to be responsible for triggering her psychotic symptoms. She concluded her report with the recommendation for an "alternate placement" for Patricia.

At this point, the meeting took on a life of its own. Instead of two factions—our side and theirs—there were really three groups. Our side was still united, but the school group broke into three parts. One was people who had met and knew Patricia. They joined our group. Then there were the people who provide special education services at the high school. Finally, there was Mr. Comstock, the Special Education Specialist. I'm not sure exactly what his role was: It was either to protect Patricia's rights to an education in the "least restrictive environment," as mandated by the Americans with Disabilities Act, or it was to save the school district money by keeping her within the local high school environment.

As we went around the table, each person who knew Patricia would say something insightful about her and recommend the kind of environment they thought would be appropriate to address their concerns. Next, Mr. Comstock would ask the special education providers at the table if they had such an environment within the school. They would reply, "No." Then he'd ask if they could invent a program to keep Patricia within the school. They would answer that they didn't know how to do that. This went on. For a long time. Patricia spoke. Her parents spoke. The guidance counselor spoke. The DMH case manager spoke. The nurse spoke. What they talked about was a kid who was so unstable she couldn't remain in a regular classroom without becoming overwhelmed within a short period of time. And each time this happened, it took a great deal of time and effort to put her back together. They just weren't set up to do that. They were all busy educating kids.

The meeting boiled down to this: Everyone at the table was interpreting "alternate placement" as "out-of-district therapeutic school," except for Mr. Comstock, who was trying to interpret it as some other setting within the existing high school.

Finally, it was Dr. Fitzgerald's turn. She said, "I've been a doctor for 25 years. In all that time, Patricia is the sickest child I have ever treated." *Ugh.*

The meeting ended.

We all went home.

∞

The school writes the IEP. I knew that. But I also knew that the family has the right to accept or reject it. And if you reject it, everyone just goes back to the table to figure out what to do.

Later that day, I wrote this email to Mr. Comstock:

BY EMAIL
From: Patricia's Father
To: Barton Comstock
Cc: Brenda Harris
Subject: Patricia IEP Thank You

November 13

To: Mr. Comstock

Thank you for your efforts to coordinate today's meeting to discuss an educational plan for our daughter Patricia. We look forward to reviewing an IEP to address her academic needs.

Later today, Patricia met with her psychologist and psychiatrist. Each feels very strongly that Patricia needs a smaller, therapeutic school environment. They do not support the idea of trying to establish something within the school. They feel she needs an established, proven program.

As you develop the IEP, we ask that you give consideration to these assertions:

☐ *The DMH psychiatrist recommends a therapeutic day school.*
☐ *Patriot Medical recommends a therapeutic day school.*
☐ *Debra White, her therapist, recommends a therapeutic day school.*
☐ *Dr. Goodman, her psychiatrist, recommends a therapeutic day school.*

- [ ] *Dr. Fitzgerald, her pediatrician, recommends a therapeutic day school.*
- [ ] *Her DMH case manager recommends a therapeutic day school.*
- [ ] *Your school psychologist recommends an alternate placement.*
- [ ] *Brenda Harris, her guidance counselor, acknowledged Patricia's shortcomings and the school's limitations.*

Because you said today that you do not have a psychiatrist or social worker on your team, unless you can provide compelling proof that these experts are wrong, we intend to rely on their professional opinions as we consider the IEP.

We believe Patricia needs a comprehensive and intensive program designed for children with psychiatric needs. And we believe her disability is one that requires her educational plan to accommodate her emotional difficulties in order for her to learn.

—Patricia's Father (with help from my sister)

∞

The next morning, Patricia sent this email to Mrs. Harris:

BY EMAIL
From: Patricia
To: Brenda Harris
Subject: Therapeutic School

Dear Mrs. Harris,

Thank you very much for the meeting yesterday. I personally feel that another school besides Abenaki High would be in my best interests. I think this because Abenaki is very big and over-stimulating, I need teachers who can help me set limits on myself, and I want to be in a situation where I will be okay asking to take a break.

I have problems in crowds, and I have known this for a while. I also seem to have trouble with different people in every class. My middle school was much smaller, there were about seven hundred twenty kids in the school, and only one hundred students had the teachers I had, and we all had the same teachers. I'm not quite sure how that helped, but I'm pretty sure it did. It's tough for me to be in a class where I don't know anybody, even by the end of the year. Last year I didn't actually meet any new people in my Math and Latin classes.

I have trouble setting limits on myself because I am an overachiever. I am never satisfied with my work, especially when I no longer have the energy to fix the problems. In a perfect situation I would have teachers whose job it was to help me with setting these limits. I can't expect this from any of my teachers at Abenaki because it's not their job and they aren't trained for it.

I try to be just like everyone else and I always feel that if they can complete a project on time or complete a test within the time block then I must be able to also. I know that I have extra supports, but I try not to use them, which sometimes puts me into even more of a pickle. If I was put in a school where everyone had these extra supports put in then I would feel more comfortable using these supports.

Many people yesterday said that I should go to a therapeutic school, and many people said I shouldn't. That's kind of a letdown because I expected the people with experience in this topic to have all the answers. I have never been to a therapeutic school so I don't know what it's like, but I feel that if this year and last year coming back to Abenaki is/was stressful enough to land me in the hospital then I should be somewhere else.

—Patricia

She wrote it herself. It was her own sentiments. I didn't ask her to change anything before she sent it.

Within a couple of days, there was an IEP. It called for an out-of-district placement at a therapeutic day school. This is exactly what we wanted. And this is exactly what normally takes a team of lawyers and educational advocates years to pull off. Patricia did it in one meeting.

Having an IEP that calls for a therapeutic school is different than actually going to a therapeutic school. First, the parents and the district need to agree on a school. Then the school needs to be willing to have the kid in their program. Finally, the school needs to have an opening. It's a little like sweet-talking the planets into aligning.

Choosing a school was the first issue. We didn't know anything about therapeutic day schools. And we already knew that the school district, with all their special education specialists, didn't know where to find or manufacture the right environment for Patricia's special needs. Our friends at DMH had only one suggestion, The Steuben School in Westford, but they acknowledged that they didn't have a lot of experience successfully placing children like Patricia at day schools.

We did some quick research on The Steuben School. Google and our ever-growing list of contacts concluded that it's an academically challenging school geared for smarter children. But it's in Westford—nowhere near where we live. In fact, the bus ride would be nearly 40 minutes each way.

Massachusetts has a system for approving private schools for special-needs children. They publish a book and operate a website, *www.spedschools.com*, listing more than a hundred certified schools and the kinds of populations they serve. I was surprised to find the website nearly unusable. Sure, I could put in our zip code and request a list of schools for kids with anxiety or depressive disorders, but selecting a therapeutic school is more about who you don't want to be going to school with than the other way around. There wasn't a way to ask the website for all the local schools that don't cater to fire setters and sexual predators.

For 10 bucks, they sent me a hard copy of the book. It took just a couple of minutes to cross out all the inappropriate schools in the state. That left me with just five possibilities. The Steuben School was one of them. Two others were local, but still nearly as far. The rest were hours away. The Steuben School was looking better and better. Maybe a 40-minute bus ride wasn't so bad after all. Our local school district was so big that some kids were on the bus for nearly an hour each way, just to get to their own high school.

Within a few days, we received a letter from the special education liaison with a list of three schools she wanted us to visit. Thankfully, The Steuben School was one of them.

We made an appointment to see the first one, an alternative high school in Leominster, 30 minutes from home. We met the director and spent a couple of hours touring the place. As was true of all of our new connections, we went through Patricia's story, trying to be as honest as possible, no longer reluctant to paint her world in its true light. We needed real solutions to real problems. These prospective schools needed to know what they were getting themselves into.

The director spoke positively about their program. She was particularly proud of their success with conflict resolution and peer mediation. Those sounded like code words for glossing things over after the hoodlums knocked out each other's teeth. Something didn't seem right.

One highlight of the tour was the wood shop. I was jealous. I want those machines in my cellar—they were just what I needed to make my new dining room table—if the lumber ever dried. The instructor spoke passionately. And the students in the room were focused and engaged. Too bad Patricia was terrified of my table saw. She wouldn't get near it.

The next highlight was the time we spent in a tenth-grade English class. The teacher greeted us enthusiastically. She spent several minutes talking almost fanatically about the real learning going on with her students. She rushed over to her desk and pulled out a big three-ring notebook. She explained to us that each year, *Time Magazine* publishes an issue highlighting their choice of Person of the Year. And each spring, incorporating everything the students have learned during the year, she asks them to choose the one person they admire the most and write three paragraphs showcasing that person's accomplishments. Pictures and artwork are encouraged. She flipped through page after page of reports, pausing at one of her favorites, one on Michael Jordan. I had to remind myself this was a class of 10th graders, not 10-year-olds.

As the teacher spoke, she was focused and engaged. On us. She gave us her full attention. What she missed, however, was what was going on around her in the classroom. It was as if she wasn't even in the room. One girl spent the whole time fidgeting in the coat closet, looking nervously into a mirror, adjusting her makeup. A couple of the boys sat at their desks, heads down, never stirring.

This did not seem like a place where Patricia could thrive.

The next school we visited was in Gardner. A couple of miles closer, but still a good trek. This was a program in search of a demand. It was housed in one corridor on the second floor of an office building. Office brick—not school brick. They look different.

Classrooms were little conference rooms, stark white paint, decorated with a white board on one wall. Filling the room were white plastic tables—the folding kind—ones you might use for a wedding or a fancy picnic outside. What was missing were students. We met a couple of teachers. They seemed friendly, and there must have been some learning going on someplace, but more than anything, it was empty, white space.

Patricia was anxious in a crowd, but that doesn't necessarily mean she would thrive in emptiness.

This didn't seem right. I started to worry.

Finally, we visited The Steuben School. It was just another 15 minutes past the last one. This place was in another office building. Still brick, but not as sterile. It was on the first floor, around the back of the building, a parking lot to itself. A basketball hoop, a volleyball net. Dumpsters, one for recycling cardboard. A snowplow blade. Somehow, the feel was different. More intimate. Better.

We met with the director, Becca Corbitt, in her office. She listened to what we wanted to say about Patricia's story, but she wasn't really interested in talking about it—she'd already read the file—she knew everything she needed to know. Becca wasn't fazed by any of it.

A new person let herself into the room. "My name is Sherry. What's yours?" *Patricia.* "Not Patti? Or Pat?" *No. Patricia.*

Someone had joined our meeting. Apparently her name was Sherry. She was talking to Patricia. Not to us. Remember one of Patricia's goals for school? "I want to be included in the decision-making process." Up until this moment, ever since she was discharged from the hospital, Patricia had been glued to her parent's sides. Sure, she was following us to these school tours, but she wasn't really involved. She was shut-down. Just like she had been for more than a year. She hadn't really been talking to anyone. With the, "Patricia," and, "No. Patricia," Patricia started participating in the decision-making process.

Sherry asked Patricia if she wanted to go with her to see some of the classes. "No." See that? Again—Patricia taking charge. It took a while, but ultimately, Sherry unglued Patricia from us and went off to see the school. We didn't need to. We weren't thinking about going there. Patricia was. On the way home, I asked Patricia what she thought of the place? "It's OK." *And do you think you might like to go there?* "Maybe."

That's all it took. Patricia participated in the decision-making process. Patricia told the special education liaison she'd like to go to The Steuben School, please. She said fine. Spring semester starts in late January. That was weeks away.

∞

In her effort to be a high school sophomore, so far, Patricia had managed to attend school for 10 days. Then we had that hospital business. Then the finding a new school part. There was a Physician's Statement for Temporary Home or Hospital Education. This piece of paper, about as effective as a written Safety Plan, entitled Patricia to a tutor several times per week, one who would serve as a conduit between Patricia and her teachers, one who would help Patricia keep up and complete the first half of her sophomore year, all without actually being in school.

We saw the tutor a couple of times between November and late January. The schoolwork, what there was of it, dribbled in from the teachers to the guidance office. Every once in a while, I would pick something up or drop something off. Patricia was able to complete everything asked of her, but there really wasn't anything more intense than writing a couple of paragraphs about someone you idolize. Brenda Harris assured us Patricia was getting school credit for all of her effort.

Patricia was not comfortable entering the building at her now-old high school. She was content when I made the trips alone. There was one trip I asked her to make with me: The one to clean out her locker. Because of all the school construction, Patricia had been sharing a locker with another student. I wasn't qualified to go down there, break into Patricia's locker, and bring home just her stuff. So we went together. School was still in session. We stopped in the office and got a pass. As we walked the halls, several students recognized Patricia and said a pleasant hello.

When we came to the main stairway by the gym, there was a big group of kids coming down. From within the crowd came this exclamation: "Patricia! I thought you were dead!" Patricia did her best to smile and nod hello. At least it was said in an enthusiastic tone rather than one of disappointment. Later, in the car, I asked Patricia about the girl who had shouted from the stairs. Patricia said she wasn't surprised that she was the one who would say such a thing. More than a year later, this same girl joined Patricia at The Steuben School as its newest transfer student. Patricia wasn't surprised about that, either.

∞

Overall, Patricia was doing quite well. Certainly not perfect, but much of the panic and sadness was manageable. She was still reading profusely. The vampire books weren't around yet, but Patricia managed to choose books just as bloody. They were giving her nightmares. Patricia had too much time on her hands and was reading too much. As a big fan of reading, this was not an easy conclusion to reach. But I decided Patricia needed to be busier. The only real question was how to go about that. We were already going to every appropriate movie a couple of times every week. We went to our favorite museums. Again. And again.

School. That was the answer. We'd try a little home-schooling. I must confess this is something I'm not trained for. And it turns out to be something I'm not very good at either. My approach was to try to turn some of the school assignments into extended projects. Maybe I could get her to focus on something for a couple of days rather than the small handful of minutes she traditionally needed to complete nearly any assignment.

Patricia was taking American History. I hated history. I mean I really hated history. But apparently I didn't hate it enough to move out of Massachusetts, the Cradle of Liberty. It turned out that much of the stuff they were trying to teach Patricia actually happened within an hour's drive of where we lived.

Field trip! Maybe we'd find some dioramas.

The assignment was to write a pamphlet, one of those two-page newspaper-like things written by rabble-rousers just before the Revolutionary War began. She had to write a couple of stories and at least one advertisement in that style. We got into the car and drove east. Boston's that way. First stop was the Bunker Hill Monument. It's this big obelisk to commemorate a battle named after the wrong hill. We climbed it. Then we went to the affiliated museum. Apparently no one goes to that museum—they just climb the monument and then head off to dinner in The North End. We went up the stairs, around the corner, and there they were: Dioramas. I was on cloud nine. But this was supposed to be about Patricia. And school. And pamphlets. So I did my best to avert my eyes and be more cognizant of the other things in the museum. It was missing two important ones. We already know about the first: Other visitors; it was just us. But the second thing missing was staff. We needed a docent, one of those retired gentlemen who tell the stories of the exhibits, one who the young children-visitors sometimes ask if they were actually at the Battle of Bunker Hill. No such luck.

Patricia followed me back to the entrance to find the guard who let us in. I asked him if he had any examples of the pamphlets that had instigated this moment in history. He gave me a blank stare. I recognized the stare—Patricia knew how to do that when she didn't know what else to do or say.

I asked again, this time substituting the word "newspaper" for "pamphlet." I saw a little glimmer of understanding. But that's different than actually getting the answer. He picked up the phone and called Joe. "Joe, this is Bill from the museum. Do you have any idea where to find examples of pamphlets—you know, newspapers—from Revolutionary times?" Pause. "OK. Thanks." Click.

He suggested we go to the Boston Public Library. "They have all the original stuff over there." *Thanks.*

Off we went.

The library was cool. Big. And stone. And imposing. Like a vault. Like a safe place to keep the things we were looking for. We asked at the desk. Pamphlets from Revolutionary times. Newspapers. "Oh. Down and to the left, up the stairs to Microfilm." *Thanks.*

"We" found another desk and asked the lady. "We" means that I asked the lady while Patricia stood behind and to the right of me, looking a little bit like the guard at the museum. The lady was very helpful. She showed us, on her computer, how to access the online database of each of the major pamphlets published in the 1770s. She directed us to a computer and had us sit down. She warned us their public computers were a little slow and we might be much happier doing this from our own computer at home.

We spent a few minutes snooping around on their computer. Everything *we* were looking for—excuse me, everything Patricia was looking for—was there. The only problem was that it really was too slow. The lady was right, this was ridiculous. We got in the car and went home.

It occurred to me, as we were driving home, that not only was it ridiculous that the Boston Public Library's computers weren't fast enough to access the information they contained, but it was ridiculous that after going to the actual places where the history happened, places charged with keeping a record of that history, places that operated an entire tourist industry based on that history, and once we were actually interested in learning something about that history, they would send us home to look it up on the Internet. If that is really the right way, why would anyone ever come out from under the covers and get out of bed. The laptop computer works just fine under there.

When we got home, Patricia spent a couple of minutes online looking up some pamphlets. And then she spent a couple of minutes making her own pamphlet for history class. Done. Back to sitting around at home. Waiting for school to start.

The characters returned for the first time since the hospital.

My attempt at home schooling was a disaster.

∞

School started.

The spring term started on a Monday. Patricia was invited to start the previous Tuesday. They had a couple of new students starting on Monday. Coming early would not only ease her into school in a slow, controlled, and safe manner, but it also meant she would be the new kid for only four days. After that, the Monday kids would have that distinction.

Patricia went to school just for the afternoons on Tuesday and Wednesday. She added lunch on Thursday. Friday was her first full day. By Monday, she was already a part of the school community. Wow, apparently, these people had done this before.

It took a while for me to figure out how this new school worked. Patricia was going. Not me. And they didn't tell me everything. The bus would pick her up early in the morning and drop her off mid-afternoon. I'd ask how her day went. "Fine." It was a little like talking to Beth (in a good way). And her schedule didn't make a lot of sense, either. There were classes with names like "group" and "academic support."

It became clearer over the next couple of months. Patricia had a head teacher, Gail, who also happened to be her English teacher. Her job was to understand and be responsible for Patricia's academic progress. That didn't mean she had to do the work for Patricia, just help her understand what was required and see that the work was completed. That used to be my job. Patricia also had a clinician, Tara, who was responsible for her emotional health—another one of my jobs. I was beginning to like this place.

Sherry was the head of clinical services. That meant if Tara was out sick, someone else might be around to rescue Patricia. It turns out that the place was crawling with clinicians and teachers who were eager to help … any time.

Andrea was the nurse. She had a school full of emotionally fragile kids and was pretty good at figuring out whether the problem was physical, emotional, or some combination of the two. She'd either send Patricia home; or to see Tara.

Becca, the director, kept it all together.

It turned out that it was just like a regular school, except with a few differences. One of the important ones was that families were actually encouraged to communicate regularly with the staff.

Cool.

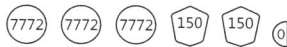

+ (4359) + (4359) + (4359) + (FLAX))) + (4359) (4359) (4359)

+ (4359) (4359) + (125) + (125) + (0) (0) + (100) + (832)

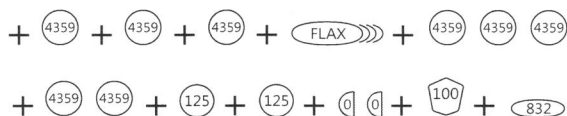

A Therapeutic School

Patricia came home from her first real day at The Steuben School. *How was it?* "OK." So far, so good.

Then she asked for her PRN. Ativan. *Why?* "Anxious." *How long has that been going on?* "Since the bus ride home … when I saw the police car lights … maybe longer." *OK.*

Time passed. Days. Then weeks. And then months.

We still needed to work on keeping Patricia engaged. Like that time at Abenaki High, Patricia wasn't coming home with very much homework. What there was could be completed during academic support, her first class in the morning. "Academic support" is code for "study hall," except there really was a teacher in the room who was eager to provide support for academics.

Monday and Wednesday afternoons were filled by CEC, the Consortium Enrichment Classroom. This was a DMH-funded program offered to Patricia as part of her eligibility for their services. A van picked her up shortly after she got home from school and drove her to the program space in Worcester. Some days they made cookies. Or a piece of art. Maybe a trip somewhere. There was time for homework. When the idea of this came up, I was skeptical. Of course Patricia's anxiety went off the charts. *Do you want to go see the program?* "No." *It will be fun. You'll like it.* "No." *Please?* I persisted. When she finally agreed to check it out, I thought we'd end up with a train wreck when she got home. *How was it?* "Fine." *Huh?* "It was fine."

The after school program services kids from age 10 through 16; after that they kick you out and make you go to the young adult group. There were two CEC sessions. Patricia was in with the older ones. These kids were all DMH clients with emotional and/or mental health issues. Remember how Patricia had trouble with other children when they act like children and don't follow the rules? What better breeding ground for trouble than a bunch of kids with a mental health diagnosis? But she had a great time. It turns out she wasn't in a group of wild and unruly brats; she was with a bunch of kids who were trying their very best to cope and deal with the challenging hand life had dealt them. She fit right in. She liked them. They liked her. It was unbelievable.

Tuesdays were filled with appointments. Deb at four every week—when she didn't cancel—and some weeks, Dr. Goodman later in the day—every two or three weeks when things were going well—every week when things weren't.

∞

I tried to talk Patricia into taking the Dialectical Behavioral Therapy course again. "No."

I tried to talk her into taking a teen stress-reduction class. "No." *Please?* "No." *It will be fun. You'll like it.* "No." When I finally talked her into checking it out, we went to the orientation. I spent my few minutes talking with the facilitator—explaining that this was not some ordinary stressed-out teenager—there was more going on. "OK." When Patricia finished her session with the facilitator, she was crying. She had a headache. Telling her she didn't need to go to the stress-reduction program didn't make the headache go away. It took a while to figure it out, but it turned out Patricia had mono. When I was a kid, that landed you at home for a month. Now-a-days some schools let you come to school. The Steuben School had a strict "No PC" policy, no "personal contact," so neither the kids nor the teachers were ever allowed to touch each other, anyway. She was welcome.

But this headache episode uncovered a chink in the perfect armor The Steuben School was using to protect Patricia. One day, she got a headache at school—no surprise—she had mono. She asked her teacher if the nurse was in. This was her way of saying, "I want to go see the nurse because I have a headache and I need some Tylenol." The answer was that the nurse wasn't in. So Patricia sat in class and suffered with her headache for most of the day. Midafternoon, as school was finishing up, Patricia managed to figure out that others at the school are authorized to dispense Tylenol when the nurse is out. Good to know for tomorrow. The next day, she had a headache again. So she modified her approach for the teacher. This time, she said, "I have a headache. I need Tylenol, please." The teacher called up the nurse and left a message saying Patricia had a headache and needed some Tylenol, please. Near the end of the day, Patricia learned the nurse wasn't in, so no one got the message. I was pleased Patricia was creative enough to change her approach when the first attempt failed. But I worried when she suffered for an entire day every time things didn't work out.

Ultimately, getting 11 1/2 hours sleep was the trick to making the headaches go away.

I did talk Patricia into taking a glass blowing class. It kept her busy for a couple of hours each week for several weeks as she formed white-hot molten glass into flowers and vases and drinking glasses. She almost threw up during the first class, but she made it through. Nerves. Anxiety. In the end, she had a good time. And she acknowledged that the satisfaction of accomplishing something was worth enduring the stress that went along with doing it. Sitting at home under the covers might not have made her feel worse, but it certainly never made her feel better. Functioning in the world with how badly she was already feeling wasn't working out at all well, so making things a little worse, now, in the hopes of satisfaction later, seemed worth the risk. As the father, it was my job to bring up these ideas.

It made me feel like an arsonist.

∞

Destination Imagination was in full swing again this year. I was managing Beth's team. Patricia was with her old team from Abenaki High. They had started late, so she didn't really miss anything by being in the hospital. Meetings were once a week, increasing in length and frequency as the March tournament approached. Patricia's teammates were worried about her. She was more distracted than last year. The team spent a lot of time designing their skit so it could work either with or without Patricia. They didn't want a repeat of last year.

They lost to Monson. Again. No real surprise. Patricia made it through the day. Incredibly, Beth's team went on to state finals. It was a good year for everyone.

A few days later, the characters came back. Voices. Out of the blue. They were from Monson. But unlike the real kids from that town, these characters weren't very pleasant. But unlike last year, Patricia did not end up in the hospital. We saw the same building anxiety in the weeks before the tournament, the same strength and resolve during her performance, and the same bursting bubble and letdown in the hours following it. The only thing missing was adding James at the last minute. But that was only because the team had pre-planned to make that eventuality unnecessary.

∞

Tara called from school. The characters showed up there, too. They were around for about 5 minutes of every 15. They were talking among themselves and also directly to Patricia. They weren't telling her to do anything; they were just talking at her. Patricia recognized the voices, but she couldn't identify whether they were the voices of some of her friends or just previous characters. Apparently she could no longer tell the difference.

Patricia reported being a little depressed. Joy was missing from her life. But she reported being safe. "Are you safe?" was a new question we asked from time to time. Patricia answered honestly. Sometimes I didn't like the answer.

Tara said she had tried to call Deb. Her voicemail picked up, but the mailbox was full. This had been happening more and more frequently. Unfortunately, we knew this because it was becoming more and more necessary to alert Deb to Patricia's latest adventures. Tara said she would call Deb's office and leave a message with the staff. Sometime last year, Deb moved her practice from Lee Street Family Services to Sinclair Health, another, larger, group practice. We just went to another building. The only things that changed were an improvement in the quality of the reading material, the seats in the waiting room were more comfortable, and the parking was free. I was happy. Patricia didn't notice any difference. Except that Deb was out sick more often.

Patricia had a good birthday. She smiled for the first time in a year.

We spent a few days in a kind of shaky, nervous calm. It was a great relief from how things had been going.

It didn't last for very long.

Instead of a call from school, this time I got an email. The voices were interfering with Patricia's ability to focus in class. She was having racing thoughts. The characters were talking about car crashes. Patricia was 16 and now old enough to drive. Even Patricia could see the connection. The fact she chose not to think about driver's education or getting her license didn't mean she couldn't still obsess about it.

As we got into May, school was starting to wind down. There were only a few weeks left in the spring semester. Patricia was a welcome member of The Steuben School community. She had a couple of friends. She ate lunch with people. She came home and told us stories of the daily exploits of multiple classmates. She was lonely. But not completely alone.

Kate and I visited with Tara about once a month to swap stories. Emails and voicemails flew back and forth. Patricia really didn't know it, but the entire school staff worked together every day to keep track of, and guide, each student's emotional (and educational) journey. If something was going on at home, I kept the school informed. If something was happening at school, I heard about it from them. That doesn't mean we were living Patricia's life for her, or even guiding where it was going, only that we were all there to nudge her back on track when things got unsteady. A little like the bumpers at the bowling alley.

∞

Family friends in town announced that the every-once-in-a-while cruise to Bermuda was on again for this year. Did we want to go? We'd done this several years ago. Our first cruise. The one with Brian and his family.

Patricia would be in school this summer for the first time. The Steuben School operates year-round. Students get a week and a half off at the beginning and again at the end of the summer session. Some kids take a week or two off during the summer, but the school districts frown on it. (Because they end up paying a lot of money to educate and bus a kid who is not there.) And anyway, The Steuben School discourages extended time off for first-year kids. The cruise was scheduled during a time Patricia needed to be in school. Not only that, but Patricia still wasn't in any shape to step onto another boat after the fiasco two years before. Patricia would not be cruising this summer.

However.

Kate announced I was taking Beth. Beth and I would go without them. They would stay at home. Kate would get Patricia up and send her off to school. For some reason, I agreed to this. When the time came, Beth and I had a great time. Friends on the boat were fun. And for the first time in two years, I wasn't sleeping with one ear open. I had forgotten what it was like to actually relax. I even felt safe enough to have a beer. I hadn't had one of those in years. The highlight of the trip was a moped ride to the bridge at Whalebone Bay, an hour after the full moonrise, to watch the fire worms fluoresce as they swam beneath us. It helps to travel with the son of a biologist—that shore excursion wasn't on any cruise ship's itinerary. Beth would never have experienced that if we had waited for her sister to get better. Neither would I.

And Patricia got to spend some quality time with mom, who was finally putting her stroke behind her.

∞

Patricia's treatment team kept getting bigger and bigger. We had all those "psy" people: Psychiatrist, psychotherapist, primary care physician. But we also added an endocrinologist and a dietician. Patricia was still gaining weight. They blamed it on the medicine. Their solution was to add even more. Flaxseed Oil this time.

∞

School ended. For a week and a half. Then the summer session started. From my perspective, nothing really changed. I still had to get up at some ridiculous hour, make Patricia breakfast, and pour her onto the bus. Patricia was dutifully taking her meds at 7:00 at night, falling asleep by 9:00, and sleeping until 6:50—nearly 10 hours. But she was still exhausted in the morning. Patricia invented something called the "bus nap." Like sheep, "bus nap" can be either a singular or plural noun. And like sheep, there were usually more than one. Patricia would take her shower, have breakfast, lie down on the couch, and crash. Sound asleep. She programmed her watch to automatically wake her up 30 seconds before the bus showed up. She'd stagger to the bus, and then fall asleep for the hour ride to school. Once there, by the end of first period, Patricia was usually awake enough to be considered a member of society.

School was a little different in the summer. Mornings were academic classes. Afternoons were allocated to off-campus intern programs or something fun at school. Patricia was presented with a list of possible internship opportunities. Nothing was promised, but there were options such as shelving books at the library, helping with the animals at a local farm, picking vegetables at another farm, volunteering at a veterinary clinic, or being an assistant counselor at a summer camp. Patricia likes animals. She chose helping with the farm animals. But that fell through. Then she chose the camp. That fell through, too. So she chose the vet.

Bad idea. Really bad idea.

Patricia's job at the veterinary clinic was to hang out with the doctor. Straighten up the examination space. Be with the animals during the examination. Hold the dog's paw during surgery. And just stand there and watch as the doctor euthanized the sickest patients. Lucky thing Patricia didn't have an anxiety disorder. It could have gone really badly.

Oh, wait.
She did.
It did.

One day, Patricia came home from her stint with the vet and apologized to our dog for getting it fixed all those years ago. Thankfully, the internship wasn't for the entire summer. Just two weeks. Everyone knew things were going badly, so Patricia was given the option of ending the program after the first week. But we know about Patricia and school. Of course she went back for the second one. As that week ended, Patricia was offered the chance to extend the program for yet another week. Apparently, the vet really liked her, so the offer was made—something that didn't happen very often. Patricia thought about it. I was very proud of her when she said, "No. Thank you. I've had enough."

I was also proud of her because she made that decision herself. The school and I watched for a couple of days as she thought about it. We talked behind the scenes and decided it would be best if she worked it out on her own. Her anxiety level skyrocketed. She sought out Tara at school. And for the first time ever, she realized it was OK to be miserable at her school and not flee for home. Lots of kids have bad days. Lots of kids at The Steuben School have bad days. And The Steuben School has the supports necessary to make it a safe place to be a kid and have a bad day.

Being a vet had always been on Patricia's short list of things to do when she grew up. It got crossed off that summer.

The voices came back again.

Deb chose that week to be sick again.

But Dr. Goodman was there. He added more medicine. The new side-effect was sleigh bells. Patricia knew all about ringing in the ears. But this was different. It was like Santa was on his way. But unlike the real Santa, who only works one night per year, these bells went on for weeks without letting up.

School ended again for the week and a half before Labor Day. We managed to squeeze in a family vacation for all four of us. Sometimes, it's just important to take a vacation from being ill. Mickey was very nice.

∞

School started again in September. Her junior year. Although she'd only been out of school for 10 days, the start of the new term counted as a transition. Historically, Patricia had trouble with these. She had landed in the hospital after the previous two September school-starts. We had hoped the continuity of the summer school program would mitigate the anxiety associated with the beginning of the fall term. But change is change. And change was Patricia's breeding ground for her anxiety. New kids on the bus. A slightly different pickup time. A new schedule. New teachers. New classes. Gym … for the first time in a year. The anxiety grew. And festered.

Patricia was proud she made it a year without a hospitalization. But I was remembering Deb's comment about how the goal wasn't necessarily to stay out of the hospital; the goal was to actually be better. Could you actually be a bad parent by successfully keeping your kid out of the mental hospital? That doesn't seem right either.

The characters were around much of the time. They were talking about fatal car crashes involving mom. And fires. Patricia was extremely distracted by them.

Time to try another anti-psychotic medication.

This one's side-effect was that she couldn't think or read or do her homework without the characters interrupting her with their stories. One of them was considering suicide. Patricia began to report a desire to harm herself. She wasn't contemplating suicide, yet. And that was only because she thought she could get the relief she needed just by cutting herself. But this is where her logical thinking breaks down. Because she didn't cut. And therefore, she never got the relief she craved.

Unless she found pleasure in the feelings associated with needing to cut ... but not cutting.

Dr. Goodman said it was time to start considering ECT, Electroconvulsive Therapy. This scared me even more than the meds.

∞

Although Patricia was in a new school, we weren't done with the old one yet. Patricia and I had spent a lot of time doing things and going places over the past year. She had used her high school student ID to get discounts on many of these activities. I "encouraged" (code word for "forced") Patricia to ask if she could get a student ID from The Steuben School. They said they didn't have one. So I called the special education department at Abenaki High. After a bit of checking, they decided they would be willing to issue Patricia an Abenaki student ID. Technically, she was still enrolled there. And technically, she was entitled to all the rights and privileges of any other student. That meant she could go to the prom, the football games, or attend any other student activities. It also meant she was entitled to have a student ID.

All Patricia needed to do to get one was to show up at the high school on photo day to get her picture taken. We decided to go early in the morning, after the high school started, but before her school began for the day. I could see the anxiety building as we drove closer to Abenaki. Walking in the door was tough. Stopping by the office for a pass was even tougher. Explaining to the photographer she didn't have a homeroom number was even worse. Actually taking the picture went fine. Driving to The Steuben School afterward was better. But when it became clear we were a few minutes late for the start of her school and Patricia would miss part of her first class of the day, the anxiety came rushing back.

Being the driver and the witness to all of this doesn't necessarily make me any smarter. Sometimes I don't come to the obvious conclusions, even when they are staring me in the face:

1) Stay away from Abenaki High;
2) Don't miss school.

∞

We knew we had a sick kid. So far, she'd been hospitalized four times. She was in a therapeutic high school. Every day she continued to struggle. But she wasn't stuck in a rut. It was more like a bumpy road. Because every day something new came up.

College, and what to do about it, becomes the overwhelming issue for most high school juniors and their parents. But what do you do when your child has some "issues" that might interfere with the parent's hopes and dreams for their child's future? Give up now? Ignore it and steam ahead? Proceed cautiously? We were still new at this. We picked "Ignore it and steam ahead."

SAT tests are a rite of passage for students thinking about going to college. Most kids take them in the spring of their junior year. Patricia had been taking high-stakes test for several years now. Massachusetts has the MCAS tests, the Massachusetts Comprehensive Assessment System; she needed to pass them in order to graduate from high school. Although the tests were anxiety-provoking, Patricia still managed to do OK. She would pass. But once again, she was doing better in math than in English. This was contrary to everything we knew about Patricia's strengths. I thought maybe it had something to do with her test-taking skills.

I decided Patricia would benefit from taking an SAT prep course. They teach test-taking strategies, provide opportunities to take practice tests, and attempt to take the mystery and anxiety out of the experience. Abenaki High offered the course as an after-school program. Patricia was welcome to sign up. I talked her into it (code for "made her do it").

The class was once a week. It started at 3:30. Patricia didn't get out of school until 3:00 and the drive was 45 minutes, so the only way Patricia could make it in time was to leave The Steuben School during the middle of her last class of the day. I called Tara. Everyone talked it over, including Patricia and her teacher. Patricia was having absolutely no trouble in her class—I think her average was 104% at the time—and she was only going to miss part of one class and only once each week, so everyone agreed that leaving a little early was not going to be a problem. Patricia heard and agreed to this. And because the SAT Prep Course was really school-related, leaving school early to go to school wasn't really leaving school early. Patricia heard and agreed to this as well. I got to drive.

It turns out the agreeing to do something and actually doing it are two different things. It turns out that agreeing that leaving school a little early isn't a big deal and actually not stressing out about it are two different things. And hearing that she'll still graduate after missing a little bit of school and actually believing it are two different things. It also turns out that rationalizing that there is not anything wrong with going into your old high school and actually not freaking out when you drive up are two different things, as well.

∞

Near the end of September, Patricia came home from a bad day at school. Instead of paying attention like a good student would, Patricia had spent her whole day thinking about different ways to cut. She'd already demonstrated she knew how to do that, so I wondered why she'd wasted her day working on that. But she's pretty creative. Most of these were new ideas I hadn't heard from her before. And most of them involved simple, household items that weren't locked away in the medication safe. For example, breaking a plastic spoon would generate a sharp edge.

We headed off to EMH again. As usual, it took more than 12 hours of anxious waiting to talk with someone who could help. No matter how bad the waiting room is or how long it takes, just the act of being there, away from home, away from school, and away from the certainty of tomorrow's same-old-schedule, changed Patricia. She felt better. When it was time to talk with the screening psychologist, Patricia was able to say that although she had an urge to cut, she had no intent to cut. And although she wanted to be dead, she had no intent to attempt suicide and therefore was not going to kill herself.

Those words got Patricia home that night rather than admitted to the hospital. It was really late, but she got to go home. They sent her off to talk with her own doctors and therapists: Those who know her best. The only problem with that is those same people had been trying to figure out what to do, without success, for the last couple of years. Just because their patient landed in the hospital last night isn't going to make them any smarter or more focused on the need for a solution. They already knew there was a problem and were trying their best to address it.

Patricia got the day off, and then went back to school the next day. To prepare for this, Patricia and I talked. We did it quietly at home, because there wasn't a hospital bed to sit on.

The goal was to figure out what to say to the school. After these trips to the hospital, The Steuben School asked for a meeting to talk about what happened and to ensure Patricia was safe enough to come back. We made a list. This is what she came up with:

Things to Talk About with School

- ☐ *I am anxious about the SAT prep course.*
- ☐ *I am anxious about being at my former school.*
- ☐ *I am anxious about missing the last few minutes of school to get to the SAT prep course on time.*
- ☐ *I am anxious about not getting credit for the class I'm missing because I'm leaving early to make it to the SAT prep course.*

☐ *I am anxious about not having enough credits to graduate
high school because I missed some classes because of the
SAT prep course.*

☐ *I am anxious about missing the education I would have
gotten had I not missed those classes.*

☐ *I am anxious about the prospect of the day coming that a
teacher tries to teach me something I don't already know
and understand. (This had never happened. Yet.)*

Notice the words. Some phrases show up regularly: "SAT prep course" is one. But the other is "anxious." We knew about anxiety. But we never really knew just how all-consuming it was.

Dr. Goodman upped the meds again. By now Patricia was taking more pills each day than the number she took the first time she committed to suicide. But things weren't better. They deteriorated. The suicidal ideations were back. And all-consuming. Now she had a plan: antifreeze again. And if she had some, she was prepared to drink it right now. After a while, the fact that she didn't have any, and therefore had no plan to act, didn't matter. Within the week, she ended up at the hospital again. Before we left, I printed out Patricia's medication log, a history of her ups and downs over the last couple of years, and Dr. Barnes's treatment recommendations. I stashed them in my pocket, so they wouldn't end up locked away when we got to the hospital.

We sat in the waiting room from late afternoon until near midnight—a record short wait—to get screened. The psychologist knew Patricia from a previous visit. This time they decided to keep her. And this time, unlike the previous four placements at Patriot Medical, they wanted her admitted upstairs, in Six West, the psychiatric ward right in this same hospital. I asked why not the Children's Psychiatric Unit at Patriot Medical again? They blamed it on the insurance company. When Patricia was 13 and 14 and 15, Patriot Medical had the contract to care for those psychiatric patients from our town. Now that she was 16, East Side Health was responsible for treating her, and they usually did so in Six West, the hospital's adult psychiatric unit.

Adult? Patricia isn't an adult. She's 16.

They sent a runner down from upstairs to get her. It took only slightly less time than it normally took for the ambulance to come that would have driven her across the state. He handed me three pieces of paper to sign. They were the typical forms: Consent to Treat, Consent to Bill my insurance company, and the Voluntary Committal for a psychiatric evaluation.

I knew about these forms. We'd signed them all before. I was OK with the first two, but the last one worried me. It gave the hospital the right to hold Patricia for three days, even if she or we wanted her out of there. I was worried they might put her in with a bunch of psychotic, out-of-control lunatics. Oh wait, Six West is where they lock up the psychotic, out-of-control lunatics.

So instead of signing the forms, I decide to ask one question. "With the patients you have on the unit now, is Six West a safe and appropriate place for my 16-year-old daughter?"

The guy looked at me a little funny. Apparently no one had ever asked this question before. I wondered why. He gestured at the forms. I asked again. He decided it really wasn't necessary to sign them down here. They could wait until later.

We trooped upstairs. I was expecting a wheelchair, but they let Patricia walk.

The door was bigger and sturdier than the one at Patriot Medical. No wire-reinforced glass. Just door.

We stepped inside and were ushered to the consultation room next to the nurse's station. One of the staff came in and asked what the problem was with the forms. He had the air of being in charge. I asked my question. He thought about it and then explained that Six West was a unit for patients 16 years of age and above. He said Patricia would have a room to herself. And he said the unit is a safe place for a 16-year-old. He handed Patricia the three forms and asked her to sign them. Patricia looked to me.

I had one second to make my second important decision of the night. I nodded. I knew the only appropriate form for Patricia to sign was the Voluntary Committal form; the others were still for just the parents until the kid turned 18. But I decided not to stop it. I figured it was OK that Patricia signed them all, just as long as I got to sign them too. *Big mistake*. As Patricia signed each form, she handed it back to him. When she was done, he gave me the

Voluntary Committal. I signed it. He took it, turned, and walked out of the room.

Linda, one of the nurses, came in a few minutes later and took over. She started handing more things to Patricia for her to sign. There were a bunch of Release of Information forms. One for her therapist. One for her psychiatrist. One for school. One for DMH. And one for her parents. I asked why there was one for the parents? Linda said that without it, the hospital couldn't talk to Kate or me. This didn't seem right. Next was a Health Care Proxy. Patricia asked me what that was. I did my best to explain it.

Bells were going off in my head. This wasn't right. Patricia was 16. None of this was appropriate. I thought about standing up, taking Patricia by the hand, and walking out. But we'd already signed the Voluntary Committal form. And there were locked doors in the way. And Patricia wasn't safe anywhere except in an appropriate hospital. I wasn't about to take her home. And I was fairly sure the hospital might decide to use their clout to reveal me to the world as the bad parent I really am.

I remained seated.

And then I asked about what they had in mind for a treatment plan. Linda said that beginning in the morning, Patricia would be meeting with one of the hospital's adult psychiatrists, a social worker, and other hospital staff to develop a plan. Then, with Patricia's permission, it would be implemented. In a few days, Kate and I might be invited to a discharge-planning meeting.

Klaxon horns were going off in my head. Terror flashed in Patricia's eyes. This wasn't right. She was 16. I told Linda this.

She moved on, as if she didn't hear me. Linda wanted to know from me whether Patricia would be safe by herself on the unit or if she needed a one-on-one aid to keep an eye on her. Without thinking, I blurted out the right answer: Patricia would be safe. Then I asked if it would be possible for someone on the staff to spend some time with her in the morning to help her get acclimated to the routine. Linda explained that aides are an all-or-nothing proposition, so that would not be possible. Instead, she called to a patient out in the hallway, one who happened to be walking by, and beckoned her into the room. Linda asked her if she would be willing to look after Patricia in the morning. She said, "Yes," and shuffled back out the door.

Even more of those bells were going off. Patricia looked panic-stricken.

So I asked about how school worked. Linda said there is no school or teacher, but there would be time available during the day for Patricia to do any work provided by her school.

Linda was done. I was done. The papers in my pocket—the medication list and history—had never moved. I encouraged Patricia to call me and talk if she didn't understand any of the recommendations the hospital made. I stood up and walked out. Someone unlocked the door for me. Had I done anything else, I'm convinced I would have been arrested. I also knew that walking out was the wrong thing to do. The problem is I had no idea what the right thing was.

I drove home. It was two a.m.

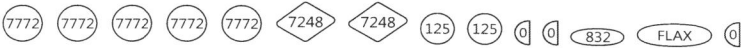

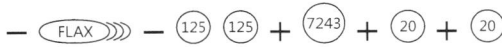

— (FLAX)>> — (125) (125) + (7243) + (20) + (20)

The Dark

The Internet doesn't sleep. Neither do I. So I got to work.

Nothing I heard at the hospital made any sense. I'd been to enough parent support meetings and seminars to know something wasn't right. The hospital was treating her like she was 18. As the kid begins to get close to 18, she gets to participate more and more in some decisions, but it's still my insurance. And it's still my kid. Kate and I couldn't be out of the loop yet. And Patricia was too busy being sick these last couple of years to be spending a lot of time thinking about how she was going to manage her illness on her own when she became an adult. It was too soon. She didn't need to do that yet. *Or did she?* And another thing: I always thought that once she turned 18, she was still welcome to include us, or others of her choosing, in her treatment decisions. That's not what I heard tonight.

Within a couple of hours, I had convinced myself Patricia didn't need to be an adult quite yet. Some 16-year-olds do, but they are not the norm. She wasn't married. Or in the military. She hadn't convinced a judge to kick her parents out of her life. Patricia was just a regular kid. I looked up all the lingo on the Internet and wrote a letter. I wasn't sure who it was for, but I did know it needed to get somewhere. Fast.

I finished my letter at seven a.m. At two minutes past, I called the office of the hospital ombudsman. The hospital's website said you could talk to them or your nurse about protecting your rights. I got an answering machine. I wasn't willing to wait around for a couple of hours for no one to call me back. So I called the nurse's station on Six West. Gary answered the phone. I asked for the head nurse. He said I was talking to him.

I read him my letter. It was only one page. I ranted about Patricia being a minor, all those forms she shouldn't have signed, their lack of a child psychiatrist, and the wealth of knowledge we, as Patricia's parents, had that the hospital didn't seem interested in incorporating in their treatment planning.

Remember Brenda Harris from Abenaki High? She was the guidance counselor who made that sound when I called to tell her about the computer sending Patricia that letter? Well, Gary was making a sound too. It wasn't very loud, and maybe it really wasn't there, but it sounded to me like he was croaking out a weak, guttural groan as I spoke each sentence. Like he was squirming in his seat, overcome by a primordial tick. He was very respectful. He listened to everything I needed to say.

When I was done, he thought for a moment and then responded. He said everything I said was correct. That Patricia should not have been treated as she was. She should not have been asked to sign those forms. She should not have executed a Health Care Proxy. That, as parents, we must approve all decisions. That another adult patient should not have been assigned to show her around. That they do in fact have an educational component. That, although the normal treatment team does not include one, they regularly consult with adolescent psychiatrists. And, finally, that Patricia should not have been promised a single room to herself—she might end up with a roommate—if an appropriate match comes onto the unit.

He agreed to pass my comments along to the social worker.

I asked him to have someone tell Patricia she was not on her own.

I went to bed.

Kate and I met with Patricia and the social worker early that afternoon. He had heard my concerns from Gary. As we talked, it became clear this was all news to Patricia. I could see a wave of relief flowing over her. Apparently Patricia had spent the night and entire morning thinking she had been cut off from her familiar support mechanisms. I expressed my frustration that they never got back to Patricia last night. He apologized to me (not Patricia) for the misunderstanding—he didn't exactly agree they did anything (or everything) wrong—but he *validated* (a DBT term) my anger. I made a point of handing him a nicely printed and signed copy of the letter I had read to Gary earlier in the day. He accepted it. And then he asked me if these events had so severely damaged our relationship with the hospital that we wanted Patricia moved elsewhere.

Wow.

That was an interesting gesture.

But Patricia was already in a hospital staffed with the kind of doctors she really needed. And they had promised she would be safe. What more could we ask for? But the real question was, would Patricia be better off somewhere else? The only thing I knew for certain is that there were plenty of places they could send Patricia where she would be significantly less well off.

I asked Patricia what she thought. She shrugged. I agreed that this was an OK place for her to stay.

The hospital psychiatrist came into the room. He said that he had lots of experience treating adolescents, he had already consulted with their child psychiatrist, and they had some ideas they wanted to try during this hospital stay. In the meantime, he wanted Patricia to stop taking Flaxseed Oil. Apparently it can aggravate psychosis in patients with schizoaffective disorder.

∞

Six West was different than the Children's Psychiatric Unit at Patriot Medical. It was calmer. What was missing were all the little kids running around and arguing with the staff. Everyone here moved a little slower. Patricia was the youngest on the unit, but there were a couple of other teenagers. And unlike Patriot Medical, where Patricia's room was the place we spent our visiting time, Six West had a strict rule that visitors were not allowed down the patient-room hallways. I think this was to protect the privacy of all the rock stars, politicians, and other celebrities who might be lurking down there.

So instead of setting up residence at the end of Patricia's bed to have our quiet conversations, we found a table in the common room. There were always lots of people around, but they either talked quietly among themselves, watched TV over in the corner, or drifted from here to there. There were street clothes. And there were bathrobes. There were patients who looked like punk rockers gone bad, those who looked like college professors, and others who looked like corporate executives. It was a nice, comfortable place. Everyone looked welcome.

Patricia did her best to adapt to the routine.

The next day she told me about the Sensory Room. I didn't get all the details, but it seemed like a place with lights and sounds and touch. It made her feel at one with the universe. She seemed brighter. And happier. And relieved. She asked if she could go home.

Not quite yet.

The next morning, things weren't quite so good. She had figured out this was an adult unit. "Why aren't I in an adolescent facility?" And she was now disappointed with the groups. She said the squeaky wheels got the grease. She was here, too. "Just because I sat quietly in the corner during group didn't mean I don't need some grease, too." She was disappointed the staff didn't do more to engage her. I encouraged her to say something. She said she'd try, but she also gave me permission to pass her comments along to the staff. I did.

The characters were still around. Although the doctors were starting to tweak her meds, nothing was kicking in yet. I asked her what the characters were saying today. She told me.

For the first time. Ever. Here's the story:

TODAY'S STORY

Sarah giggles as she combs her fingers through her blond, sweaty hair.

SARAH — to Jay: "It's really too bad Drew's not in our gym class. Today was so much fun."

DREW: "What did you do this time?"

JAY: "Soccer ... with a bouncy ball."

SARAH: "More like pinball, bouncing off us."

JAY: "Lots of fun."

Drew, Jay, and Sarah are best friends even though they each belong to a different clique. After school that day, they each went to hang out with other friends.

DREW'S MALE FRIEND: "Look what I got!"

DREW'S FEMALE FRIEND: "Cigarettes?"

Drew didn't smoke.

DREW'S MALE FRIEND: "Better! I got my hands on a gun."

ALL OF DREW'S FRIENDS: "How?"

DREW'S MALE FRIEND: "Why, you know I trust you all, but a guy's got to have secrets."

DREW'S FEMALE FRIEND: "So, whatcha gonna do with it?"

DREW'S MALE FRIEND: "Who'd deny a dare?"

They all looked at Drew. They were all tough. He was soft in comparison.

DREW: "What are you all looking at me for?"

They handed him the gun with a dare to shoot someone that night. Drew goes outside after dinner. He sees someone walking in the woods nearby, aims, and pulls the trigger. He recognizes the scream. It's Sarah's. By the time he reaches her, Sarah is limp. She doesn't respond.

DREW'S MALE FRIEND: "You really did it! Awesome, man."

DREW: "I just killed one of my best friends."

DREW'S FEMALE FRIEND: "She's a loser and no good for you. It's better off this way."

DREW: "No, it isn't."

Drew walked away, thought for a minute, then came back and tried to smile.

The next day at the school bus stop, as Jay and Drew and other bus kids are getting on the bus, only Jay heard Sarah's voice.

SARAH, also getting on the bus: "Jay, why do I feel so weird. I was walking in the woods and something hit me. I woke up there and now nobody can see or hear me."

JAY: "Sarah, I'm hearing things. You got shot. You're dead!"

SARAH: "I don't feel dead ..."

JAY: "I can't see you. Only hear you."

FIRST BUS KID — to Jay: "Dude, you're talking to yourself!"

SECOND BUS KID: "That kid in the paper is your friend, isn't she?"

JAY: "Yes, Sarah is my friend."

JAY — to Sarah: "AND SHE'S DEAD!"

Unable to see Sarah, one of the bus kids sits down in the seat where Sarah is sitting. When he moved right through her, Sarah admitted something was wrong. Drew didn't hear her voice either, and Jay was alienated.

After school, Jay and Sarah went to Drew's party. Sarah was listening in on one of Drew's friends' discussions.

DREW'S MALE FRIEND: "Simple. Get all of the crazies and losers in a car. Drive it to a freeway. Jump out of the car. Big crash. All the losers gone, just like that."

DREW'S FEMALE FRIEND: "Love the idea. Who?"

Drew's female friend started collecting four kids to put in the car. She went up to Jay.

DREW'S FEMALE FRIEND — to Jay: "This party is lame. Care to go someplace cooler?"

SARAH: "DON'T GO!"

JAY: "Sure. Sounds cool!"

Drew's female friend got into the driver's seat and drove onto the highway. She jumped out of the car. It crashed. Sarah screamed.

Jay, seemingly unhurt, emerges from the twisted, bloody wreck.

Now able to see Sarah, Jay goes to her.

Jay embraces Sarah, while they look back into the wreck — and down at his own dead body.

Patricia had this far-a-way look about her as she finished the story.

Uh-oh.

I knew that stories had been a part of Patricia's life for a long time. In third grade, when we heard her happier ones, we thought she was creative. In middle school, when they started to become more unpleasant, Patricia stopped telling us about them. In high school, as we began to learn they were a part of her psychosis, I struggled to understand what "experiencing these characters" really meant. I knew they had personalities. I knew they weren't always pleasant. I knew they interacted with each other. I knew there were stories of car crashes. I knew there was blood. I even knew there were homicidal themes. But nothing prepared me for the story Patricia told me. It was complicated. And manipulative. And devious.

I asked Patricia if she might write it down and share it with her doctors. She said she'd think about it.

My mind was racing. I needed to know more. But she had already told me everything. And I didn't want to make as big a deal about this as I really wanted to. So we moved on. Our quiet conversation shifted to getting some homework from school. I asked her what I could bring her from home. As Patricia was answering my question, she stopped and said, "Jay embraces Sarah, while they look back into the wreck — and down at his own dead body."

What?

" 'Jay embraces Sarah, while they look back into the wreck — and down at his own dead body,' that's where the story is again. It plays over and over again. That's where it is now."

I wasn't ready for this either.

As Patricia told me this story, there was no hesitation in her words—no need to pause to choose the right way to deliver each line. It was almost like a script. What she told me was a series of words, lovingly crafted to tell her story. The cadence was already worked out. It was mostly dialogue, but there was just enough narrative so I could understand the context and the setting. If it really had been the script for a soap opera, I'm sure the descriptions of the set decoration, the character's clothing, their appearance and mannerisms, and the layout of the blood-spattered crash-site and its victims would have gone on for pages. In minute detail. I'm sure Patricia had that all worked out, too.

But it was the words that were consuming her. The characters were playing out the scene in real time. She was hearing their words. And while she listened to them, she was experiencing all the other stuff that goes along with those words.

When I say I used to think the characters were "like a soap opera on television," I meant something different than what was actually going on here. There is a difference between watching a soap opera and being one. If a soap opera is playing on the TV across the room, even if the volume is blaring, you can glance away and it will go on without you. Not this. It was driving her. But it also needed her to make it go. When the voices were loud, they used every bit of her brain power to exist. If they were a little quieter, maybe Patricia had enough parallel-processing capability available to live a little bit of her life at the same time. But they could never go on without her. She's what made them real. And the more energy Patricia spent making them real, the less real Patricia became.

Real soap operas have episodes. Dr. Bob might be a jerk on Monday. On Tuesday, Ted might get cancer. By Wednesday, Lars, the new boyfriend, might kill off some minor character in a jealous rage. But all the stars of the show—the ones you get to know and care for—don't spend their time tricking each other into cold-bloodedly murdering each other. Everyone would be dead or in jail by the end of the first episode.

And real soap operas don't usually spend a lot of time in syndication, either. Once is enough. I always thought Patricia's stories were linear—with the stories always progressing forward— with today's story morphing into tomorrow's by the next day. It never occurred to me they might rerun. But this story was repeating in Patricia's head. It was running over and over. Again and again. Like a broken record.

> *Be strong.* (I said this to myself.)
> I already knew Patricia was.
> How could she put up with this?
> If it were me, I think I might just kill myself.

Let's do some math. Patricia's story took about 45 seconds to tell. There is time for 80 of those stories an hour. More than a thousand in a waking-day. A quarter million each year. Millions and millions since third grade.

This changes everything.

Until now, I haven't had a lot of experience with people with psychosis. There was that great aunt whom I'd never met. My father visited her a couple of times a year when I was young. She spent her entire adult life living a quiet existence in a private sanitarium, convinced she had mothered a child with the king of England. I was never invited to any royal events or otherwise saw any evidence this might have been true.

A couple of years ago, I read the autobiography of a young woman who grew up with psychosis. One of Patricia's doctors recommended I read her book and had told me that Patricia reminded her of this young lady. The first time I read it, I was so distracted with how the details of her life story were so different from Patricia's that I missed all the important parts about the nature of her psychosis. When the doctor mentioned it again more than a year later, I read it again. This time, I paid more attention to her account of her auditory and visual hallucinations. She talked about how there were different characters—each with their own agenda. Giant men. Faces in doorways. In windows. Even in an opening drawer. It all boiled down to the fact that they were all out to get her. To steal her thoughts. To make her hurt herself. Or others. But it still sounded like one of those soap operas. It wasn't until I heard this young lady tell her story in public, when I could actually hear the terror in her voice and see it in her eyes, that I understood for the first time just how unacceptable it must be to try to live a life while consumed with these distractions. She talked about being angry she was alive; about how she "couldn't live" for one more day with the voices—"couldn't live"—not "couldn't imagine living."

She convinced me.

More recently, I met a young teenager who was struggling with his own mental health. He was heading down a path similar to Patricia's: depression, bipolar, suicide attempts, lots of meds. And psychosis. One night, the faces of his hallucinations appeared at his bedroom window. They were after him. He convinced himself that if the lights in his room were bright enough, they would stay away. But the only light came from the nightlight plugged into his wall. And that wasn't enough. So to make it brighter, to protect himself from those very real tormentors, he took a match and lit the plastic housing of his nightlight. Just to make it brighter—so they might stay away.

He burned the house down around his fleeing family. Thankfully, they had the forethought to keep the batteries fresh in their smoke detectors.

∞

That day at the hospital, I learned the voices are real. And if they want it, they have the power—and the intent—to kill.

That day, I think I began to understand the sadness.

And the panic associated with the prospect of it coming back.

I saw the dark.

And I knew that the only way Patricia was going to survive was if we could make her voices go away.

Period.

There really wasn't any other option.

I was pretty sure that if we couldn't find a way, Patricia would.

Parent Support Groups

I went to see *Rent*. Again. It's a Broadway musical that had started touring around the country. Kate, Patricia, Beth and I had seen it in New York during its original run. I'm not really sure what it's about. Those who know more than I say it is a modern retelling of *La Bohème*, whatever that is (It's an opera by Puccini, whoever he is). But this version has something to do with love and AIDS and living and dying in New York. The music is haunting. And popular. When Patricia was in fifth grade, her school chorus included some of its songs in their holiday concert. I was always surprised the music director overlooked the words and the themes when she selected music for an elementary school performance. Or had she?

For the last couple of years, every time the show came to Boston or Providence, I found myself drawn to it. Kate and I managed to get to the movies together regularly; we could pull this off because Patricia was medicated at 7 p.m. and asleep for the night by 9. And Patricia slept so soundly, we knew she would be safe if we went to a 9:30 movie that was playing 10 minutes from home. Driving more than an hour to go to an 8:00 show wasn't something we could do together very often, so again, I ended up going alone.

As I sat there, dead-center in the eighth row, (because you can buy a single ticket dead-center in the eighth row on the day before the performance even if it's been sold out of the two-seats-next-to-each-other seats for months), I realized the story playing out in front of me was actually my life. I was Mark, the filmmaker-character in the play. He spends his entire existence lurking on the sidelines, documenting what's going on around him, as the rest of the characters, including Angel, the drag queen who succumbs to AIDS in the third act, all live incredibly full and deeply satisfying days. Mark's only contribution is to get in the way while he tries to film everything.

My favorite song in the show is sung by one of the bit-part characters, Gordon. It's less than a minute long. He sings it as he introduces himself to today's group at the Life Support meeting at the local community center. These meetings are a chance for men and women who are living with the inevitability of death by AIDS to get together and talk—to talk about whatever they want. About how they are feeling. Physically. Emotionally. Spiritually. Mark, of course, bullies his way into the meeting.

This day, at this performance, for the first time, I heard and really comprehended the words of Gordon's song. He sings about how he is surprised to be alive. How logic and reason no longer work for him. How he should have died three years ago.

We were just passing the three-year mark on Patricia's journey.

She was still alive.

I'm supposed to be the engineer. And on that day, I was having trouble with logic and reason, too.

∞

I'd been going to parent support groups for most of those previous three years. Kate went with me to the first meeting. I went alone to the next one. Years later, I still make it to nearly every one.

For my family, the idea of airing our dirty laundry in public or admitting life is anything but perfect is unthinkable. And because we tend to flee from controversy and handle things quietly on our own (think oil-burner story), we'd never find ourselves in a place where delicate subjects might even come up. But the events surrounding Patricia's hospitalizations were so terrifying—the Prozac checklist to suicide, the inaccessibility of the doctor, and the uncertainty of how to talk with Patricia's school—that I knew Patricia, and all of us, needed more protection than me and my fire extinguisher could deliver on our own.

So I went.

To listen.

Not to talk.

Just to sit in the corner and listen.

The parent partner who had originally suggested the idea of a parent support group was adamant that we go. She brought it up again after we pooh-poohed the idea the first couple of times. And when we finally said yes, she made sure we knew she had called the group facilitator to let her know we were coming to the meeting on Thursday night. So much for quietly AWOLing the whole thing. I suspect the whole process was conspired against us—because it would have been so easy not to go. (And, by the way, if it wasn't planned that way, it should have been.)

I called my mother and asked her if she would be willing to babysit Patricia, our now 14-year-old daughter, while Kate and I went out for the evening. She agreed. Kate and I drove to a nearby clinic, one largely funded by DMH, and a place where Patricia and I would spend a great deal of time at DBT training sessions and specialist appointments over the next few years. As we walked in, Judy looked us in the eye and welcomed us with a smile and by name, "You must be Kate and Bob. Welcome. I'm Judy. Find a seat. We need to feed the kids first, and then, after they go into the playroom, we'll get started with our meeting." If there was a corner, I would have chosen it—but there wasn't—so we joined everyone else at the table. We had a few bites of potluck dinner (not bad—we were new so we didn't need to bring anything) and I did my best to avoid eye contact with everyone around me. The small talk was familiar—just like a bunch of friends getting together. I've never been able to function in these kinds of settings in my other life. Tonight wasn't any different. I managed to avoid saying anything substantive until the meeting started.

The children ranged from about 6 to 11 years old. Patricia would have been the oldest. We were still new at this and I was still convinced Patricia would not have tolerated coming along. As dinner finished up, the kids migrated next door to the playroom. Food wasn't allowed in there, but that didn't prevent a lively discussion about whether cookies were permitted or not. Somewhere, these kids had learned to advocate for themselves—to participate in charting their own futures.

Wow!

Maybe Patricia could learn something from them.

Judy, our group facilitator, began our meeting with a discussion of the ground-rules:

Parent Support Meeting Rules

☐ *Meetings are only open to parents or caregivers of children struggling with emotional or mental health issues. No rubberneckers allowed.*

☐ *Everything said is confidential.*

☐ *Don't talk about anything in front of the children.*

☐ *To respect everyone's privacy, don't acknowledge others if you see them in public outside the meeting.*

☐ *Everyone gets a chance to talk.*

☐ *No one is required to share anything, just say, "Pass."*

Except for the missing secret handshake, this was a little like being the member of a fraternity. Or the Masons.

Today's meeting, just like the hundreds that followed, began with introductions. The goal is to put a name (just first names) with each face and briefly introduce the circumstances that make you a candidate for attending a meeting such as this. The process should take about 20 seconds per person. After my hundredth meeting, I had refined my introduction to something like this:

"I'm Bob. My wife Kate and I have two perfect children: Beth is the angry 12- (or 13-, or 14-, or 15-) year-old. We don't believe it, but everyone says she's developing normally. Her sister, Patricia, is 15, (or 16, or 17, or nearly 18). She suffers with depressive (or bipolar, or anxiety, and/or schizoaffective) disorder(s). She's been hospitalized two (or three, or seven) times. This week, we're working on finding a doctor (or finding the right med, or finding the right school, or getting her to sleep, or trying to wake her up, or learning Dialectical Behavioral Therapy, or coping with the voices, or trying to control the voices). Things are going badly (or terribly, or really scary, or even, occasionally, better)."

And then on to the next person. Simple as that. By doing it this way, everyone in the group gets a sense of who their audience will be today and can tailor their remarks to be most appropriate.

Kate and I were new at this. On that first day, we had no idea what to expect. Introductions were made around the table. Judy started. She told us about her family. It was clear she belonged here. The next person announced that her kid was out of control. No diagnosis. Just completely unmanageable. The next one's child was in the hospital—had been for the last three days. She thought he might be bipolar. He wasn't any better, but the hospital was trying to send him home anyway. After that, it was the parent of the girl who was a little angel a few minutes ago at dinner, but who we could now hear through the playroom wall. She was acting out in school. The school kept suspending her. But they wouldn't do anything to help her to keep focused in class. By the time they got to us, we felt right at home. No kidding. All the fears of showing up were gone. All the worries about being embarrassed, for yourself, or for your child, were gone. We knew we were among friends who would welcome us. We knew we were among friends who would be interested in hearing our story. We knew we were among friends who had stories to tell us. And we knew those stories would ultimately help Patricia on her journey.

When it was our turn, I mumbled something. I don't remember what I said. But I do remember the people around the table were focused and interested in what I was trying to say. There were smiles. Good smiles. Smiles of recognition. Smiles of familiarity. Smiles of understanding. And when there was an audible chuckle, it was a comforting signal that someone knew something important that we didn't know yet, and not that we were being ridiculed. It was very clear that, in some way, each of the people around the table had lived at least one little piece of our journey. Put them all together in one room, and you have a parent support group.

This is what a parent support group is all about.

This is why I keep going.

∞

Back when I first became the manager of a Destination Imagination team, Patricia was in elementary school. In the interest of trying to bring some order to the gaggle of out-of-control fourth-graders, I introduced the concept of the Talking Kaleidoscope. I'm not sure if it ever served its true purpose, but every time I brought it out for that year's new team, I did get a few minutes of quiet while I had a chance to share my vision of focused organization and team serenity with them. The Talking Kaleidoscope is my version of the Talking Stick, something I learned about first in Cub Scouts and later during one of those corporate team-building retreats in the early 1990s. But mine is more than just a mechanism to give the floor to just one person at a time. Whereas the Talking Stick is passed around the circle giving everyone the chance to be heard — the Talking Kaleidoscope also recognizes that each person sees the same set of circumstances just a little bit differently. If I look through the kaleidoscope and see the forest, my hope is you might look through it and see the trees.

If I were the facilitator of a parent support group, I'd bring along my Talking Kaleidoscope. Because if done right, the part after the introductions is the best part of the parent support group meeting. And it only works if just one person is talking and everyone else is reinterpreting and adding to that single discussion. Ideally, it goes something like this: One by one, each member of the group is given a chance to talk. To talk about anything they want. And they know they are entitled — and expected — to talk for their proportionate share of the remaining minutes of tonight's group — less two minutes at the end for wrap-up. It's a time to spend bringing everyone up to speed on what's happening in their family. If the group consists of just regulars tonight, then picking up from where we left the story at the last meeting is sufficient. But if there is someone new, a couple more sentences might be necessary to put everything in perspective. And if the introductions happened correctly, you know just enough about the new person to understand whether it's OK to describe last week's cutting incident as "slashing her wrists with a paperclip," or as a "self-injurious behavior." Some people have never heard of cutting — remember me? — and might not be emotionally prepared to hear something so terrifying, let alone in such a flip manner.

But the truth is that in order to get anything done — in order for the kid to hope to get any better — the parents need to get over the delicacies of what's going on with their kid and really try to understand what the problem is. And by the end of the first meeting, although they didn't know it walking in, today's new parents are ready to hear the worst—because their own version of something just as horrible is going on in their home, too.

That night, I learned I wasn't alone. That I wasn't the first parent to have a kid with some big-time problems. That I wasn't the only parent who didn't know what to do. That I wasn't the only parent who didn't have a clue about how to start doing things to make Patricia better. Up until then, it was only me, not knowing what to do to help, as I watched Patricia not know what to do to help herself.

But that night, too, I learned there were things to do. By that time, I did know that the doctors, at least the ones we were dealing with, didn't have all the answers. And I knew Patricia wasn't going to magically get better on her own. She was heading down the path toward dead, not the one toward recovery. I learned that the people in that room, or in another room like it, were my best resources to find the answers Patricia needed. And that I needed to be the one to spearhead the Second Quest. Because Patricia couldn't do it for herself.

Because she was too busy being sick.

∞

Remember how I said I wasn't sure what I said that first night? Well I'm not. And it isn't that I didn't write it down. I probably did. The reason I don't know is because I can't find my notes for that day. I probably have them. I've probably seen them as I searched for them. Back then, I didn't write in full sentences. And I didn't bother to date things. It took me a while to figure out that this was going to be a long-term project.

Where I wrote stuff down changed over time. I started with scraps of paper. After a while, I switched to a spiral-bound notebook that I jammed into my front pants pocket. It lived there for months along with my fingernail clippers, lip balm, jackknife, and pen. Invariably, the cover would come off and the first few pages would self-destruct before I got around to changing it. Finally, I ended up with a small writer's notebook. The company that makes it claims Hemmingway used one. They have a big version—too big for my pocket—and a small version—too small to actually write anything useful. So I buy the big one and cut it down to halfway in-between: 3" x 5". I reinforce the sewn spine with some bookbinder's tape. And I jam it in my front pocket. If I were smarter, I'd switch to a new one every three months, whether I filled it or not.

I try to write everything down. But sometimes I forget. More is better. Questions for the doctor. What the doctor said. How Patricia is feeling. What she said. How she looks. And if things aren't going quite right, which they never seemed to do, I try to remember what happened in the previous minutes, hours, or days that might have had something to do with today's not-quite-right. I write that stuff down, too.

The prize from all this work (which really doesn't take very long), is the raw clues to what is going on with the kid. And the parent support group is one of the times to stop, look back, and try to understand what has happened since the last meeting. I have my notes. And I can use that same place to write down my thoughts for what I want to talk about at today's parent meeting. Just the act of deciding what to say makes me think about what's been going on and forces me to make a judgment about whether it is important enough to bring up. And knowing I'll have the time to say it all at the parent meeting, unlike at the doctor's office, forces me to think about what I might say when one of my fellow parents thinks it might be important and wonders what I'm going to do about it.

Stop.

Let's repeat that.

What. I. Am. Going. To. Do. About. It.

The word "I" is in that sentence. Not the kid. Not the doctor. Not the school. I. Me. The whole point of the parent support group is to help *me* figure out what *I* am going to do about it. We already know that the kid doesn't know what to do. The doctor might have some ideas, but really doesn't know your child. Nor does the school. But maybe if *I* can point one of them—the kid—the doctor—or the school—in the right direction, maybe then something might actually get better.

This is what a parent support group is all about.

My experience is that waiting for someone else to do it doesn't work. And my experience is that if you procrastinate about doing what you've already figured out needs doing, things don't get done. And things don't get better, either. This is the beauty of the parent support group. Because whether you know it or not, if you make it through your story, and if you talk about your ideas, and if you listen to ideas from the others, and if you come to some sort of conclusion about what you might do, you will leave the meeting having made a promise to them—and to yourself—to do that thing and report back on how it worked out at the next meeting. And if the meetings are held twice a month, as they should be, you need to do something this week, so you can see how it works next week, so you can talk about it again in two weeks. If you do this for a year, and only come up with one idea each meeting, you will have made 24 attempts to improve things. And that's 24 more chances for the kid to get better than if you sat at home and waited for the kid or the doctor or the teacher to fix something.

Guess what? They aren't going to fix anything.

And your kid will suffer because of it.

∞

It turns out there are two kinds of parent support meetings. That first one was a Sharing Meeting—everyone just sits around and whines (in a good way). The other kind is a Speaker Meeting. Every once in a while, Judy invited someone to come talk to our group. As much as I missed the sharing, many of the speaker meetings were incredible. We got to talk with an educational advocate—for free—for two hours. We learned what they do, why you might hire one, and we listened to the tactics they might use to convince the school your kid needs a 504 Plan or an IEP. And we learned about some of the tactics school districts might use to write an IEP or 504 Plan that won't cost them as much as the one your kid really needs.

Another night, we talked with a psychiatrist. He wasn't there to prescribe medications, but he was willing to talk about medication strategies and to give feedback on the kinds of information that would help him as he listened to the patient or the parent. I had more time to ask him questions during that session than at five or more appointments with Patricia's real doctor. And although we weren't talking specifically about Patricia, we were talking about how to optimize our time with Patricia's doctors, so from that day on, every appointment was far more productive than it ever would have been.

The next guest specialized in testing. She talked about the differences between psychoeducational testing, neuropsychological testing and projective testing. About how each was appropriate for different purposes. But really, she talked about the importance of getting testing done so that all of the kid's doctors and therapists would be working on the same, right, things. It's almost like you can't fix anything unless you know what the problem is.

There were other speakers: Lawyers. Financial planners. Writers—of a book trying to find the humor in their messed up families. Stress reduction facilitators. And so on. Every once in a while, we'd have a guest I was convinced was going to be a complete waste of my time. I'd try to think of an excuse not to go—maybe spend some time at home talking with Patricia. Or Kate. Or Beth. But I usually went. And invariably, I'd walk out of the meeting having learned one or two new things. Things I never imagined I needed to know. Things Patricia could use, starting tonight, to improve her situation. Even things *I* could use, starting tonight, to improve *my* situation. I never regretted going to one of the meetings I thought I should skip. But I always missed the lost opportunity to share.

∞

Most parent support groups have signup sheets. By putting my name down on the list and divulging my email address, another new world opened up to me. I started getting emails. Most were invitations to more programs or groups. Some were filled with helpful suggestions. I read them all and imagined myself going to some of these events. When a parent group in Arlington announced that a couple of guest speakers from NAMI, the National Alliance on Mental Illness, were coming to their meeting, I decided to go.

Two women from NAMI's "In Our Own Voice" program spoke. They were survivors. Adults. Real people, living with a mental illness, who had managed to make it to adulthood. They told their stories. The bad parts of one sounded remarkably similar to Patricia's journey. The other was different, but horrific in its own way. And for some reason, these women weren't dead. Meeting that parent partner from so long ago was my first step in understanding that other parents have lived—and lived through—the hell I was going through. But that night, for the first time, meeting these survivors was my first opportunity to see that there might be a path through Patricia's own hell that doesn't necessarily need to end in suicide. This was amazing.

Recovery? Hope?

A speaker meeting meant it wasn't a real sharing meeting, but it still began with brief introductions. So although I didn't know the full story of the parents at this Arlington group, I did hear that many of their kids were more like Patricia than those from my other group. Sicker. I decided to come back to Arlington for a sharing meeting and check it out. I went. And went back.

Over time, I found yet a third support group. And I frequented that one, as well. Each group is different. Each has its own personality. Some groups meet at night. Others during the day. Some have childcare. Some serve pizza. Others have potluck. One group was all about camaraderie. Lots of small talk. "My car broke down. Again." Where to get a deal on the kid's underwear and socks. It seemed like this was the only time these people ever got out. As if it was the only contact they had with the outside world—both for them and for the children they brought with them. It took me a while to figure out that this was their reality.

Other groups are all business. Just talk about the kid. And how the kid's behavior is destroying the family. Those are my favorite.

I get different things out of each group. But I've found I need each of those things in my life. So I keep going to all of them.

Many of the regulars at these meetings, particularly the ones with childcare, are single parents. They don't have someone else at home to witness what is going on, to talk about it, or to strategize about what to do. For me, in order to make a decision about what I'm going to do next as I try to be supportive, my brain needs to spend some time thinking it through. But I'm not smart enough to do this on my own. I need a sounding board. Knowing I should talk at tonight's parent support meeting forces me to mull it over at least once beforehand. By the time I go through it again at the meeting, I may be ready to say out loud what I might already know. And if I haven't figured it out yet, my compatriots will be there to help me see through the fog. Most importantly, I count on them to see through my rose-colored smoke-screen and tell me when I'm full of it.

∞

Not all meetings are as perfect as the ones I just described. For me, those without structure are the worst. When we all sit around and chat for two hours, with everyone jumping in when they want, the conversation deteriorates into drivel. That's not why I'm here. I'm at this meeting to learn something useful to help my suicidal kid stay alive for another day.

Not all parents are as perfect group-participants as they could be. Some have trouble staying on topic. Others have trouble understanding what the topic even is. There is a big difference between strategizing ways to make the school understand its responsibility to find ways to help Johnny focus and complaining about being dissed by the assistant principal during the meeting that was supposed to get Johnny that help. Complaining about how the meeting went is fair game for a parent support group discussion, but except for a brief "validation of feelings" (that DBT term again), the only way to make a real difference is to move the conversation to one of what to do next. Whining isn't going to fix anything. Talking about what to do differently tomorrow, might.

Not all parents are as perfect at keeping things confidential as they could be. Every once in a while, out in the real world, I run into someone from group. But before I ever consider speaking with them, I stop myself. I look around the room. I think about where I am, I think about whom I know. And then I wonder about how many people the other person might know. If anything doesn't seem right, I make an imperceptible nod in their direction and walk away—we can talk later. I hope they do the same for me. I don't want to be with a kid or a friend or business associate, and have someone come up to me and start a conversation as if we know each other. Because once that conversation is over, I don't want to explain what it was all about: "Oh, didn't I tell you, Patricia has bipolar disorder. She's been suicidal recently. That was Natalie from my parent support group." No. Please no. I already have enough problems.

It's happened.

It's awkward.

It's dangerous.

Not all group facilitators facilitate as well as they could. Meetings should start on time. If today's meeting starts on time, the person who is a couple of minutes late might be on time for the next one. If today's meeting starts 10 minutes late, the person who showed up 9 minutes late will be 14 minutes late next time. There is no reason to waste a second of opportunity to discuss what is keeping our children from living the lives we wish they had.

And if brief introductions are part of the deal, they need to be brief. The meeting I go home most angry from is the one where a couple of parents, including me, have made our 20-second introductions, and then the next person goes on for half an hour. At that point, the meeting shifts to sharing. And invariably, time ends just when we make it around the room for the first time. Those of us who try to follow the rules and make our introductions brief never get a chance to share whatever it was we needed to talk about. And we came to talk—not to get some good-sportsmanship medal for doing what was expected. It is up to a worthy facilitator to keep us on track. We parents are so wrapped up in our own selves and problems that we can't regulate ourselves.

If we didn't need facilitators, we wouldn't have them. Anyone can unlock the door.

Properly implemented, team-building exercises integrated into the introductions at the beginning of the session have spawned nearly all of the best meetings I've ever attended. The trick is to insert a bit of chaos into the normal flow of the evening. If I'm coming to the meeting all pumped up to talk about the week's stupid IEP meeting, it's easy to start ranting about that during the introductions. However, if the facilitator says something like, "Let's go around the room, quickly. In three sentences, introduce yourself, the child who is the reason you are here, and then tell us something good they did this week," it changes everything. "Tell us something about yourself we don't already know," works just as well. Suddenly the train of thought is shattered. Everything you were planning to say goes out the window, and the need to come up with an answer to the unexpected question pushes the real agenda off to the sharing part of the meeting. Where it is supposed to be. You can learn a lot from the answers to those questions. And just that little insight is enough to make the rest of the meeting much more productive.

That is the kind of meeting I want to attend.

But the best meetings, and the ones that make them all worth it, are the ones where the facilitator (or a very brave fellow-parent) gives me a little nudge and pushes me just slightly outside of my comfort zone. On a good night, it happens just at the end of my turn, right after I've said my piece, right when that incredible feeling is just starting to kick in:

I'm done. I'm ready to go home.

By showing up and talking, I've fixed me.

But I'm there for Patricia … and she's not fixed, yet.

What comes next is usually in the form of a simple question: "What are you going to do tomorrow?" Or, "You shouldn't feel like a prisoner in your own home." Even, "How does that make you feel?"

Like a sledge hammer, the serenity is broken. Whereas a second earlier I was ready to put it all behind me, instantly, tonight's problems come right back to the forefront. Dread floods. Then panic. Because the only answer to whatever the question happens to be begins with an "I," again, and involves promising to do something: "I'm going to call the school … or the doctor … or my DMH case manager." Or: "I can't continue at this pace … I need some sleep." Even without a concrete plan, just admitting I need to get some sleep greatly increases the chance I will figure it out and get it done.

This is why I go to parent support group meetings.

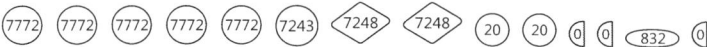

− (7772) + (50/902) + (7242) + (50/902) − ⟨7248⟩ ⟨7248⟩ − (7242)

− ⟨0⟩ ⟨0⟩ − (20) (20) − ⟨832⟩ − (50/902) (50/902) + (CG596) (CG596)

More Junior Year

Patricia came home from the hospital on not one, but two antipsychotics, Clozapine and Risperdal. Risperdal is the older version of Invega, the first medicine that gave Patricia some relief more than a year ago. And the one Dr. Barnes said wouldn't work.

But the combination did.

The characters were gone.

For a while.

Patricia was feeling better. School welcomed her back. We invited friends and family to Thanksgiving. They came. Kate cooked a great meal. We all ate at the new dining room table, the one I made out of the tree from the front yard. After three years, Kate was back to cooking for a crowd, the lumber was finally dry enough to use, and I had a few evenings of peace (and not quiet) in the cellar with my table saw and new thickness planer. It would take another couple of years to put the final coats of finish on everything, but it was a start.

I wish things were going better with Beth. The day we got home from our "Newfoundland" trip, we weren't a quarter mile from home before Beth and Patricia were squabbling again in the back of the car. And everywhere else. Beth was sick of having a sick sister. She was done pretending to be accommodating. Instead of walking around on eggshells, she started shouting. When I tried to talk with her about it and asked her to be more understanding, she said, "The things Patricia has so much trouble dealing with are no different than what everybody has to put up with. She should just get over it."

But maybe mental health is all about the struggles of not being able to get over it.

After the holidays, Patricia's anxiety started to build again. It began at school. She was the only one in her math class. One student. Some kids would hate this; no way to disappear into the background. Others would love it; the undivided attention of the teacher. Patricia, of course, found it insufferable; she needed others in the class to struggle with her as she was introduced to some difficult concepts—things, for the first time in a long time, that she didn't already know. She needed others to come up with the questions she didn't think to ask.

A little voice inside me reminded me that Patricia was in the most advanced math class offered at her school that year, probably ever. And, as a junior, the chance of anyone being in next year's even-more-advanced math class was nearly impossible. The voices inside Patricia's head were talking about car crashes. And, for the first time, Patricia was one of the fatalities in their stories. It became clear that there was only a limited window before things were destined to deteriorate. In the past, we spent a lot of time appreciating how well things were going and we'd wait for the world to start crashing down around us before thinking about what to do next. Planning for disaster takes up valuable time that could otherwise be spent living, but because *not* living was still so high on the list of possibilities, I decided to plan ahead.

The first call was to the psychiatrist from East Side Health, the one who had just tweaked her meds. I thought he might be interested that his brilliant plan to get rid of the voices had only worked for two weeks. Maybe he had a suggestion about what to try next. It turns out he wouldn't see Patricia—because she wasn't an inpatient in his hospital. If she wasn't sick enough to be in the hospital, then she wasn't sick enough to rank him. This didn't make a lot of sense to me. I hope you see the flaw in this, too.

Dr. Goodman was being his slow and methodical self. "Give the meds a chance to work. Patience." But when the urge to cut became unbearable again, he added yet another medicine. And that made Patricia look overmedicated again. "Drugged into a stupor" is the picture I want to paint.

She started reporting bizarre dreams again: She was attacked by a stapler. Her braces fell out. I (dad) was mad (about the braces).

I got a call from the school nurse. Patricia showed up in her office with a racing heartbeat for no apparent reason—pulse of 130—had we ever seen this before? Yeah, she was already taking a drug for that. I guess it doesn't work, either. Patricia sat quietly and self-soothed herself back down to 88 within 10 minutes.

Even though Dr. Goodman wasn't helping, he wasn't against another second opinion. I made more calls. I called East Side Health again. Did they have any other doctors who would be willing to see Patricia? No. They only do inpatient.

I called Mystic Valley Healthcare. That's where Dr. Barnes got us started on the campaign to get rid of the voices more than a year ago. She wasn't available; she'd been hired to head the child psychiatry department of some other hospital and was in the process of moving to Worcester.

Mmm.

They didn't have anyone new doing adolescents.

Now that Deb was hooked up with Sinclair Health and their network of child psychiatrists, maybe she had a suggestion of where to get a consult. I asked after one of Patricia's erratically-weekly sessions. She gave me the name of a practitioner in Boston who specializes in Omega 3 therapies. Isn't that Flaxseed Oil?

I called my contact at the Department of Mental Health. She asked around and came up with nothing.

> Sometimes, it seems that having connections merely gives
> you more opportunities for people to say no.

During Patricia's annual physical this year, I was lamenting to Dr. Fitzgerald again about how badly things were going and how difficult it was to find someone for another idea. She asked why I didn't contact Dr. Barnes again. I explained that she had just moved to Worcester and would soon be starting her new career in charge of child and adolescent psychiatry at East Side Health Center. This was not an acceptable excuse. I explained that I had already been turned down by them.

Dr. Fitzgerald didn't care. She wanted me to contact her anyway.

I started typing:

Bob Larsted

A Quiet Street · Holden, Massachusetts 01520

508 555-0196 · bob@boblarsted.com

November 20

Dr. Sharon Barnes
East Side Health Center

Dear Dr. Barnes,

Welcome to Worcester.

Dr. Fitzgerald, my daughter's pediatrician, recommended that I write you.

Patricia suffers from difficult-to-treat schizoaffective disorder. We came to see you at Mystic Valley Healthcare last year. We credit your advice, the good work of a dedicated team, and the best therapeutic school anywhere with keeping her alive since then.

Unfortunately, Patricia's auditory hallucinations have broken through the boatload of drugs she now takes, including both Clozapine and Risperdal, the two medicines you recommended.

We are seeking a medication consult with someone who has the experience to help an extremely sick adolescent.

Our efforts to find such a person have been unsuccessful. Mystic Valley says they no longer see adolescents. We've been unable to get in to see someone at East Side. The psychiatrist who treated her recently at Six West in Worcester is the kind of professional we are looking for; but he doesn't see outpatients. Even DMH doesn't have any ideas.

Although we are pleased with Dr. Goodman's medication management, it seems ridiculous that my daughter needs to be hospitalized before she has access to someone who can help us with the big picture. But even then, once she is discharged, access to that professional is cut off. I'm not sure how many more times my kid is going to put up with being hospitalized before she is dead.

I hear that East Side Health Center has the smartest adolescent psychiatrists in the world. But what good are they if they can't treat the sick children that live in the community?

Any advice you can give us on how to access services at East Side, or anywhere, would be greatly appreciated.

Sincerely,
Patricia's Father

I spent a lot of time writing that letter. I decided I needed to share it not only with the doctor I was trying to win over, but also everyone else who had already said no. And some others. So I sent copies to:

- [ ] *Dr. Fitzgerald, the pediatrician.*
- [ ] *Dr. Goodman, the psychiatrist.*
- [ ] *Deb, the therapist.*
- [ ] *Tara, the school clinician.*
- [ ] *The psychiatrist at Six West who wouldn't see Patricia.*
- [ ] *The psychiatrist I'd met at that parent support meeting.*
- [ ] *The president and CEO of the hospital.*
- [ ] *Patricia's Department of Mental Health case manager.*
- [ ] *The local director of Child/Adolescent Services for DMH.*
- [ ] *The DMH psychiatrist who did the IRTP evaluation.*
- [ ] *The president of my health insurance company.*

Three days later, Dr. Barnes called. Three days after that, the DMH psychiatrist called. And then, my insurance company called to see if everything was OK. Actually, by that time, Patricia was back in the hospital.

∞

This is the point in our story when I should be telling you about how everything started falling apart. But instead, it's just about the time everything started going right. The DMH psychiatrist visited

Patricia in the hospital. Dr. Barnes sent one of her students, a "fellow," a post-graduate doctor pursuing additional specialty training, to do a complete psychological workup. The hospital discharge-planning meeting was the best one ever. The DMH psychiatrist came. He had visited Patricia in the hospital. He introduced the concept of "Worry." Worry is a little different than anxiety. Being anxious is something you are. Worrying is a job. A devotion. A life skill. It takes work. Being creative makes you a better worrier. It's something you can compulsively obsess about. Did I ever tell you how creative Patricia is?

Patricia's new psychiatrist at Six West came to the meeting, too. Her contribution was to add a third antipsychotic medicine. Patricia was already on Clozapine, the gold standard of antipsychotics, and Risperdal, another popular one. The third one is Navane, an older medication. Patricia would take one Navane, twice daily, but also have the opportunity to take another pill, as a PRN, up to twice more daily, if the voices returned.

It worked.

Patricia came home.

The characters were gone.

For a little while.

Then they came back.

Then she took the Navane PRN.

And they went away again.

When they came back again, she took another pill.

And they went away again.

∞

We rescheduled our appointment with Dr. Barnes. I sent her all kinds of information before we met, including an updated medication history and a blow by blow description of all the gory details of everything that had happened since we last saw her. I'm not sure if any of this was helpful, but Dr. Barnes had an ace up her sleeve. Her fellow, the one who had spent all that time with Patricia in the hospital doing the psychological assessment, was sitting in the room when we showed up. She had been able to witness Patricia's mood first-hand.

Patricia was open and honest. She answered all of Dr. Barnes's questions. Except one. Patricia had trouble answering whether she felt "sad" or "empty." I thought it was "sad." Patricia said she thought the real answer was "empty." We had to think about it for a couple of days. I asked Tara, her clinician at school. She said "empty." Definitely. "As if something is missing." She spoke of how Patricia brightens right up when someone recognizes something good about her. But she also remarked at how quickly Patricia is able to come up with something new to worry about once the previous worry is over (and turned out well). Deb agreed. Unfortunately, my "sadness" answer was based on the few times I have seen Patricia lose hope. A wave of sadness rolling over her; how she just wants it to be over; how she doesn't really want to kill herself, but how she really wants to be dead.

Dr. Barnes sent us a report a few days later. It was another one of those things a parent doesn't want to read. In the recommendation section, it suggested using Clozapine as the primary antipsychotic; reducing the Risperdal, slowly; keeping the Navane daily and as a PRN for voice-breakthrough; and adding a another, different, antidepressant to address the perhaps obsessive basis of cutting. And it recommended cognitive behavioral strategies to address the anxiety and enduring psychosis.

Patricia's diagnosis changed today. It now is:
Schizoaffective Disorder, Depressive Subtype
Generalized Anxiety Disorder.

Notice that the "Rule Out" is gone from the General Anxiety Disorder. *Yup, she has it.*

Just like a lot of kids in her class.

But they, like Patricia, had found the right therapeutic school.

∞

Plate tectonics is responsible for creating some of the most beautiful scenery on earth. But it also takes incredible destruction and a mountain of trouble to get there. Our two competing continents were the school and Dr. Goodman. And like continents, each was doing their own thing, minding their own business, and trying to make the world a better place.

The school was doing a career inventory on Patricia. Schools do this to convince their students there might be more career choices than fast food or mowing lawns. Patricia tested positive for several life opportunities.

She scored very high on humanitarian and accommodating jobs. Humanitarian jobs include occupational therapist, social worker, physician assistant, and physical therapist. Some accommodating jobs are waitress, flight attendant, and hairdresser. They also inventoried her aptitude to find out how challenging her career choice should be in order to give her the most satisfaction. She scored very high in her verbal and spatial skills, which indicates she could succeed in the scientific world. Some of those jobs include engineering, biologist, physician, and veterinarian. *Uh oh.*

The school looked at this and concluded Patricia was capable of going to college and getting a master's or doctorate degree. Then they took a look at Patricia, the kid who had been going to their school for the last year, and decided she might be happier with a BA. They talked up the humanitarian jobs because they felt the accommodating jobs were beneath Patricia's capabilities.

Dr. Goodman read Dr. Barnes's report. Then he looked at Patricia, the kid who had been coming to see him every couple of weeks for the last two and a half years, and decided that school was responsible for much of Patricia's symptoms. He recommended that she remove herself from the stressor. Perhaps get herself a GED online instead.

This is how the Rocky Mountains were built.

Rather than dismiss Dr. Goodman's school comment as the ranting of a madman, Patricia tried to give it some careful consideration. It was hard. She talked with Deb. She pleaded with me, with eyes like a sad puppy, wishing this wasn't even on the table for discussion. She talked with Tara and the career counselor at school. Collectively, we all decided that Dr. Goodman really was mad.

Patricia started a list.

And when she was ready, she told him:

Things to Tell Dr. Goodman

- ☐ *I'm not done learning.*
- ☐ *I want to graduate high school.*
- ☐ *I want to go to college.*
- ☐ *I want a "real" high school diploma rather than a GED.*
- ☐ *I want to graduate with my class at The Steuben School.*
- ☐ *I want to graduate at the same time as my other friends.*
- ☐ *I love my school.*
- ☐ *I can't imagine how some other school could be better.*
- ☐ *My school has the supports I need.*
- ☐ *I'm willing to work to manage my anxieties.*
- ☐ *Now that the voices are mostly managed, this is a good time to try to improve school.*

∞

We invented a new activity, "Fleeing." It's a coping skill. They didn't teach it in Dialectical Behavioral Therapy, but it's really a hybrid of the distress tolerance techniques we had learned in that class. When Patricia wasn't feeling right, instead of sitting around at home being miserable, we got in the car and went places. When Tara called to say Patricia was freaking out and had had enough for the day—please come get her—I picked her up and we went somewhere. We spent a lot of time at the science museum. We saw a lot of movies. And we burned a lot of gas.

The chief complaint was the urge to cut. When the characters came back, Patricia took a pill to make them go away. When the urge to cut overwhelmed her, we fled.

And fled.

My skills as an activity director leave quite a bit to be desired and I was running out of fresh ideas.

I tried to talk her into joining a young adult group with some of the DMH kids who had aged out of the after school program—just like Patricia had. They would even pick her up and drop her off at home. Patricia wasn't ready. I couldn't talk her into it. It took another six months for her youth support worker to convince her to give it a try.

Somehow, I talked Patricia into taking an online photography class with me. Over the course of eight weeks, we learned about using the advanced settings on a digital camera. Up until then, all Patricia knew about photography was holding the camera up and pressing the shutter button. Like this year's math class, everything was new to her: shutter speed, aperture settings, ISO "film" speed. Homework was due on Sunday nights. Our teacher would have constructive criticism by Tuesday.

This was a disaster.

Instead of being about learning something cool, it was exactly like school—and with all the baggage that goes along with it. There was the reading. Patricia would procrastinate about that for a few days. After that, she'd procrastinate about taking the pictures to try out what she'd learned. Then she'd procrastinate for another couple of days before selecting the images to upload for the teacher to review. By Sunday afternoon, she was a wreck—just like she was the night before any other school assignment. We'd end up fleeing, but the next week's assignment wouldn't be posted yet, so we couldn't use this time to take next week's pictures.

For normal people, getting the assignment done and handed in would signal the time for a little relief. Not with Patricia. She'd spend from Sunday afternoon until Tuesday worrying about what the teacher was going to say about her homework. As it got later in the day on Tuesday and the comments still weren't posted, Patricia would obsess about checking the website every few minutes until they were posted. And even though the teacher would always say nice things about her work, he'd also make helpful suggestions about how to make it better. For me, this was the advice I was paying for because I wanted to learn something. Patricia took it as criticism. Like she'd done something wrong.

Maybe there really was something to Dr. Goodman's suggestion.

∞

Another year had gone by. It was time to figure out what to do about Destination Imagination. Patricia had been involved now for eight years. But her team was gone. And there was no chance she could pull off starting another one with her new classmates at school. Patricia announced that her goal was to remain in the DI program—at least until she got her 10-year pin. That meant two more years. *Oh, no.* What would she do?

I spoke quietly with one of the DI state officials. I told her an abbreviated version of Patricia's story and asked if she had any suggestions. Surely this has happened before. Instead of being surprised or making some sympathetic remark, she acted as if this has, in fact, happened with other children. Her advice was to figure out something to do—anything—and stay with it. She offered to help make it possible.

Patricia made a list: New team? No, that wasn't going to happen. Be the co-manager of an elementary school team? Maybe, but finding a team that meets after school at a time Patricia could make it to from her school halfway across the state was a problem. Be an appraiser, a judge, at one of the tournaments? Maybe, but that would require a day of training with a bunch of adults, learning complicated rules, and then interacting with both adults and kids for an extended tournament day. What would happen if she freaked out like two years ago?

In the end, she figured out how to stay involved.

In addition to Destination Imagination's "Central Challenge," that eight minute "school play" the kids work on for the whole year, there is something else called an "Instant Challenge." On tournament day, each team is given a problem to solve—right now. For example, they might be asked to design a marketing campaign to encourage children to eat a newly-developed vegetable that's both easy to grow and good for you; the only problem is it tastes terrible. The team has three minutes to come up with a commercial, including song. And then they have one minute to present it. Sometimes they build things out of straws and paperclips. Other times they act out something with invisible props.

The results can be extraordinary.

Practicing all year for this type of challenge creates great learning experiences. It teaches teamwork and cooperation. It can also be the source of great stress. The first thing Patricia decided to do was to organize an Instant Challenge Day for the DI teams in our town. She borrowed the program room from the public library for a Saturday morning. For me, this day and the days leading up to it didn't make very much sense. Here I had a kid with an anxiety disorder who was prepared to stand up in front of a bunch of people. Kids. And their parents. And boss them around. For half a day. This is why we invented fleeing. But Patricia was confident enough in herself and her DI expertise that she was convinced she would be able to pull it off.

Maybe too confident. As we practiced for the day, I had Patricia try the challenges out on me. Part of the process is reading the printed challenge aloud—twice—before handing it to the team as they begin. The problem was I couldn't understand anything Patricia was saying. It was like she was talking really quietly. Really fast. With a tennis ball in her mouth. As I thought about it, this had been going on for a while. In fact, there hadn't been a conversation with her where I didn't need to ask her to repeat herself for a long time. We worked very hard to get her to slow down and enunciate. Ultimately, it worked for that day, but this was a new and persistent problem that caused lots of trouble. For a long time.

But there was something else overshadowing everything, too. The anticipation/letdown cycle was in full swing. Getting organized for Instant Challenge Day was an exercise in procrastination. As always, she left everything to the last minute. That way, she could get the high from being nervous about not being ready on time. As time ticked away, Patricia suffered from that same paralysis she got when she needed to do her homework. Everything was so overwhelming that nothing got done; she was unable to break the problem down into pieces small enough to pick one and get started. As time was starting to run out, she finally decided what she was going to do. Then, all of a sudden, she needed supplies. This provided the opportunity to worry about needing to go to the store to get them. Which provided another day of turmoil. And when we didn't go to the store right away, which would have solved the problem, we got to spend some more time worrying about not being ready on time. Driving to the store the night before, Patricia told me she was happy for the first time in a long time. She said it was like the night before a DI tournament, one filled with eager anticipation. The next day was fine. Intermixed with periods of sheer terror, Patricia managed to guide a whole bunch of kids and their managers through some great Instant Challenges. Everyone went home having learned something important. For Patricia, it was that she was able to make a difference.

A month later, on the day of the regional tournament, Patricia found a way to help out, too. She was very pleased to be able to stay involved. Each time something worked out, no matter how small, Patricia got a shot of satisfaction that she was making a difference and that she was a member of something larger than herself.

As we started home, Patricia reported having a great day. She was smiley and talkative. But at dinner on the turnpike, her mood soured. She said, "I need to cut." I asked why.

"I *need* to cut because I need to cut. I *can* cut because I don't have anything to look forward to. I wanted to do DI so I *couldn't* be in the hospital."

Ultimately, she didn't cut. But over the next few days, I saw that same post-tournament slump start to kick in. I hadn't forgotten that Patricia landed in the hospital a couple of times after a big event like this. But she was getting stronger. She made it through the week. Then another. And then another several months. Before she needed to go back to the hospital again. All I could do was watch it happen.

But over time, something was changing. The urge to cut was still there, but the medications were keeping the voices away. And for some reason, much of her anxiety. This was not like her. I decided to test Patricia's school anxiety.

In May, the winners of the state and international Destination Imagination tournaments meet in Knoxville, Tennessee for Global Finals. Although Patricia had figured out how to stay involved, next year would probably be her last one, and without a team, her chances of making it to Tennessee were slim. So I asked her if she wanted to go anyway. Just to watch. She said, "Yes."

So we skipped school for a couple of days (always anxiety provoking), got on a plane (always anxiety provoking), and immersed ourselves into a mob of more than 15,000 kids and parents (always anxiety provoking) who were having the time of their lives. We saw incredible performances put on by the best of the best DI teams from around the world, including many from Massachusetts.

I had another reason to get Patricia to go. For some kids, one of the most important rituals of Global Finals is "pin-trading." Most state or country DI affiliates create a series of custom lapel pins representing their regions and this year's challenges. Kids bring a bunch with them to Global Finals, and during the down times, they trade with each other. Imagine the hallways outside the huge university lecture halls filled with a sea of kids, each sitting on the floor with a hotel towel covered with pins, with just as many other kids strolling by, making deals, and walking off with their newly-traded prizes.

I had ordered fifty pins hoping Patricia might be willing to participate. But because we had decided to go at the last minute, and because our state had some leftovers, they sent me a hundred. Over the three days we were there, I encouraged Patricia to trade. She really didn't want to, but I persisted. Every time Patricia got a, "No thanks, I already have that one," she would feel like a failure. But every time another kid agreed to trade, she'd have that smile I missed so much. Patricia traded all of her pins. And because she had a trading success rate of about 50 percent, Patricia, the anxious kid who normally doesn't talk to anybody, initiated conversations with two hundred strangers from around the world. And even though there might have been a bit of anxiety that went along with it, ultimately, Patricia was very pleased.

How do you make an anxiety disorder just disappear?
Maybe by making the voices go away.

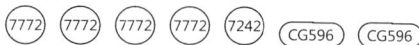

(7772) (7772) (7772) (7772) (7242) (CG596) (CG596)

$$+ \overline{\text{12 25}} + \overline{\text{12 25}} + \textcircled{\scriptsize 4359}\ \textcircled{\scriptsize 4359} + \textcircled{\tiny 50\ 902} - \overline{\text{12 25}} - \textcircled{\scriptsize 7772}\ \textcircled{\scriptsize 4359}\ \textcircled{\scriptsize 4359} - \textcircled{\tiny 50\ 902}$$

CBT Exposures

Implementing Dr. Barnes's suggestion for adding another antidepressant took some time. It was an SSRI, just like Prozac and Celexa. Wasn't it Dr. Barnes who told Patricia to stop taking the Celexa? Dr. Goodman seemed reluctant. But eventually, we all agreed to give it a try.

Patricia smiled for the first time in six months.

One of her classmates commented that she looked more alert.

She smiled for a second time. She was pleased he had noticed and cared enough to say something.

Implementing Dr. Barnes's cognitive behavioral strategies recommendation was a bigger problem. It took until after the first round of phone calls to figure out we didn't know what "cognitive behavioral strategies" meant. For a while, I expected I could just call someone and sign Patricia up. After all, that's what Dr. Barnes's report said she needed. The "someone" was the first problem. The "signing up" was the second problem.

After several conversations with Dr. Barnes's office, I finally figured out Patricia needed the CBT equivalent of a DBT course. Ideally, it would be a weekly session for adolescent females with self-injury urges. She'd learn a set of skills to target the urge to cut.

It didn't happen. If we lived in Boston, maybe. New York, probably. Los Angeles, definitely. But not Worcester. Not that I could find anyway. I called Dr. Barnes's office back. They recommended finding an individual therapist who knew CBT. I ended up calling many of those same people back. When I asked if they knew CBT, nearly all of them said that of course they did; it's part of their treatment plan. When I asked if they could teach the strategies on a short-term basis to someone with an urge to cut, they just blanked out. Clearly no one had ever asked for something like this.

In desperation, I started calling every one of my contacts. Surely someone would have an idea. Deb understood what we needed. And she knew that as Patricia's individual therapist, she wasn't the right person. I asked if she knew someone else in her new office who would be appropriate. She didn't. Patricia's Department of Mental Health case manager came through with an idea. She recommended the clinic that hosted our DBT classes and one of my parent support groups. They have a slew of therapists and doctors. Her office happened to be in their building. She told me to call the main intake number. She promised to make some back-door calls.

Within a week, Patricia was signed up for weekly CBT therapy with Dr. Kari Lang, a child psychiatry fellow from the medical school, who was scheduled to graduate in the spring. The timing was perfect. She knew exactly what Patricia needed. It didn't hurt that Dr. Barnes was one of her fellowship supervisors. Dr. Lang and Patricia got right to work.

However, within a couple of weeks, it became clear that Patricia was not getting better. She was getting worse. Much worse.

∞

Dr. Goodman added another medicine, Naltrexone. Until now, I thought I understood the rationale for each one. But not this time. Naltrexone is a drug that is normally used for opiate addicts—heroin users—for instance. It blocks the high associated with the drug, thereby taking all the fun out of being an addict. The thinking was that it would reduce the urge to cut.

This made no sense to me. Patricia hadn't cut in more than a year. How can you eliminate the rush you don't get when you don't do something? It made for interesting conversations with several doctors. The final authority turned out to be Patricia. For her, Naltrexone does not reduce an unfulfilled urge to cut. If anything, it makes it worse.

Patricia started getting dizzy. And clumsy. At home. And at school. She passed out in gym class—just hit the ground while playing tennis. She'd fall. School was getting worried. The nurse noticed Patricia had a slight hand tremor. Her teachers noticed she was having trouble focusing. After she fell asleep in sex ed class, they sent her home.

Dr. Fitzgerald diagnosed her with Postural Hypotension and recommended more fluids. And salty soup.

Dr. Goodman said the problem was the Luvox. So he reduced it. It didn't help. Patricia walked around like a Neanderthal with her jaw hanging down.

And her mumbling continued to get worse. With a couple of, "What did you say?"s, I could usually figure out what she was talking about. Same with her teachers. But everyone else in the world was having trouble. When she joined the poetry club at school, I started to worry. She had decided to read them her "Boxes" poem. It wouldn't be the same if the words were unclear.

She practiced. I couldn't understand. I tried to get her to slow down. It didn't work. I had her start reading books aloud to me. She improved, but she was still dropping the last word in every sentence and the last syllable of all the words with more than two. I didn't understand anything.

More sleep didn't help. Nothing was working. It was so bad one day that we ended up at the hospital emergency room. They pumped a bag of IV fluids into her and told her to go home, drink more liquids, and add more salt to her diet.

∞

Patricia was falling apart. She needed Deb. But Deb was sick again this week. And again next week. Maybe she'd be in this one time. But then she'd be out again. Sometimes we'd get a call from Deb or her office saying she was out today. Other weeks, we'd show up only to find that she wasn't in. Her voicemail was always full. She didn't return calls left at the office. Finally, it became clear she might not be back for a while. Or ever.

We asked Deb's office if Patricia could see a covering therapist until she returned. They acted like they had never heard of such a thing. I persisted. Finally, Donny called to say he would be willing to see Patricia. They started meeting every week. This, too, was a disaster. The first problem was that Donny spelled his name with a "y" at the end rather than an "a." Patricia announced that she really preferred a female therapist. "Donna" would have been better. Nothing personal, but it's personal.

I had a lot of practice sitting in the waiting room while Patricia went to see Deb; we'd been doing it for years. Patricia would go in at the top of the hour and stay for 50 minutes. Sometimes I would be invited in at the end to talk about how well—or how badly— things were going. It was different with Donny. We could see him through the glass at our appointed time, but he spent the first several minutes of each session rushing around from office to office in the back. And Patricia always finished early.

Patricia told me that Donny kept asking her why she was there. What was really wrong with her? Then he told her he didn't see any reason why she was on so much medicine. Patricia was coming home from her appointments very unhappy. And by the way, since when do you not need to take medication to keep the voices away, when, for the first time ever, the medication is actually helping to keep the voices away? I was intrigued by the idea that Patricia's illness could actually go away. *She'd be better?* But the problem was that she wasn't better.

The last time Patricia met with Deb before she disappeared, they decided to give each of the characters a name. Then they told them—one by one—to go away. The characters went away. And they stayed away for a long while. This was real progress. Why wasn't Donny building on these successes? Maybe it was because he didn't know the characters were still coming back now and then. Because he wasn't talking to the one who was hearing them.

Dr. Goodman was. He knew about them. And he was trying to do something about them. He adjusted her meds.

We came home one day to find a message on the answering machine from Donny's boss, the clinical director at Sinclair Health. She said they were auditing their records and had discovered that Patricia only sees a therapist at their practice. They require their patients to use one of their psychiatrists in order to access a therapist. She asked us to think about it for a couple of days and make an appointment with their psychiatrist if we wanted to keep seeing Donny.

My jaw dropped.

I fumed.

For a couple of days.

Then I called her back. I got her machine. I left a message. It went something like this:

Message for the Director

- [ ] *Nearly three years ago, at Deb's recommendation, we followed her from her old clinic to yours.*
- [ ] *We like Deb very much and credit her with keeping Patricia safe.*
- [ ] *We are surprised to learn that after all this time, something is wrong and you want it resolved this week.*
- [ ] *We believe that Deb, Dr. Goodman, and your psychiatrist need to participate in this discussion. Deb is out. Dr. Goodman is on vacation for three weeks, so,*
- [ ] *We would like to defer this discussion until Dr. Goodman returns and we hear from Deb.*

She never called me back.

A week later when Patricia went off to see the psychiatrist covering for Dr. Goodman's vacation, he told us he used to work for Sinclair Health and whenever they needed to drum up some business, they would drag out their old psychiatrist/therapist linkage policy and start making calls. He agreed that Dr. Goodman needed to participate in any conversation about moving psychiatrists or therapists once he got back from his vacation. When we went back to see Donny, he announced that because we hadn't made an appointment with the doctor, he was unwilling to schedule any more sessions and Patricia was being discharged from Sinclair Health.

I was livid.

I called the director again. She took my call this time. Apparently she hadn't gotten my message, and, no, she wasn't aware Donny had kicked us out. Although she didn't provide any details, she implied that Deb wasn't ever coming back. She acknowledged that the transition to a new therapist should be slow and controlled. She promised to talk with Donny about scheduling another appointment. She encouraged us to talk with Dr. Goodman when he got back. And she encouraged us to make an appointment with her psychiatrist.

Although I had no intention of ever going to see him, I did agree to make an appointment. We scheduled one. But he was booked pretty solid. His first opening was weeks away. *For the kid who was lucky if she made it two weeks without seeing Dr. Goodman.*

This was ridiculous. But it did buy us some time to find another therapist.

I left one last message for Deb, asking for her advice.

She never called me back. Ever. *I hope she is OK.*

After what seemed like a hundred calls, we found another perfect therapist.

One who returned our call. And still does.

∞

Patricia had been reading a lot. No matter how badly things were going, she still had a big pile of books to read. Every time the stack got small, she'd find another series. Adding books for school usually wasn't an issue; they'd just go into the pile.

Until British Literature. The assignment was to read *A Tale of Two Cities* by Charles Dickens. The problem wasn't the length—she could breeze through long books. And the problem wasn't the impossible-to-read British-English—she could handle that. The problem was that she had already read this book in freshman English at her previous school. And she hated it.

This created a huge problem. Patricia had always been compliant. If you asked her to do something, she'd do it. Not this time. Her teacher tried to encourage her. "No." I tried. "No." The other kids in the class were going on without her. Which meant she was spending more and more of her school time in Tara's office and not in the classroom. Which meant she was falling behind. So her anxiety level went up and up. Which meant I was getting more and more phone calls to come pick her up. To flee.

So much for spending time at work.

I tried to help. We sat down together and I read her a few pages—just like we used to do. It was terrible. It reminded me of trying to read her *The Adventures of Tom Sawyer* by Mark Twain when she was nine. The language was impossible. It was filled with words that I didn't know and certainly couldn't pronounce; all the characters have confusing names that all sound alike, and the storyline is complicated and convoluted. Why would anyone want to read this?

So I asked her teacher.

It turns out there is a reason:

Like *Tom Sawyer*, there are those who think it is a great work of historical fiction. It's chosen specifically because the language is difficult. In high school, teachers use this book to introduce skills on how to deal with challenging material—so the student will know how to do it on their own when they get to college. Practice for later in life. *Interesting concept.*

Her urge to cut increased.

∞

Just because Patricia wasn't doing her homework didn't keep Dr. Lang from assigning homework to Kate and me. Patricia and Dr. Lang's cognitive behavioral therapy sessions were still going badly. Apparently there are several kinds of CBT. The one they were working on had something to do with a "mood and feelings worksheet." They would talk about Patricia's urge to cut. They would fill out forms as they tried to rationalize that her feelings were unfounded.

But the problem with unfounded feelings is they have no logical reason for existing. And therefore, Patricia was unable to use logic to make them go away. She was a wreck when she came out of her sessions with Dr. Lang. Like they had just spent the last hour stirring up a hornet's nest.

Patricia suffered.

Dr. Lang asked Kate and me to be aware of when Patricia was feeling miserable and write down what we said to her and how what we said affected her mood. This is great! I'd been keeping track of this stuff for three years. Finally somebody was interested in what I've been seeing. My OCD kicked in, and within a couple of days, I had a three-page report off to Dr. Lang. I wrote everything down. Even the stuff that wasn't important. (I thought.)

Dr. Lang was ecstatic. Buried in my report on Patricia's week, she found her needle-in-the-haystack. And if I had trimmed out the unimportant stuff from that list, it would have been one of the first things to go. It was a question Patricia asked me one day when we were walking down the stairs from my mother's condo, alone, quietly chatting the way we do. She wanted to know if she might have OCD, Obsessive Compulsive Disorder.

Dr. Lang was trying to use CBT to control Patricia's all-consuming urge to cut. They had already experimented, unsuccessfully, with the rationalization variety of it. There is another form of CBT that uses "exposure" therapy to do its magic instead. It's like overcoming your fear of flying by getting on an airplane. The problem is that the cutting version of it might logically become "overcome your obsession with wanting to cut by cutting." *Nope. Too bloody.*

However.

However, counting stairs isn't.

Dr. Lang talked with Patricia about her OCD question. Patricia told her that for as long as she could remember, she had been counting each step as she climbed stairs. She did it every time; and—for some reason—she *needed* to do it every time. Same with matching the gait of people walking with her. She was compelled to match her steps with theirs. Dr. Lang asked if there were any other things like this. Patricia pondered for a moment, and then said, "Yes, I press the crosswalk button 13 times when I cross the street."

Dr. Lang was like a giddy schoolgirl. Well, actually, technically, she still was.

What she came up with was unbelievable. Once a day, for the next week, Dr. Lang had Patricia walk up or down a flight of stairs—without counting them. She could not distract herself by singing or talking to other people. She was to focus on the fact that she wasn't counting the stairs. The only other thoughts allowed into her head were these "bossing back clues":

1) It's just an obsessive thing;
2) It doesn't matter;
3) It's practice.

After she climbed the stairs, she was to spend as long as necessary just lingering with the feelings, rating them on a scale of 1 to 10, until she felt better.

Imagine if someone told you to stick your head into a bag of harmless, de-stingered hornets and said, "Everything will be fine." Would you do it? This is what it was like asking Patricia to walk up a flight of stairs without counting them. That first time, she reported being at a "7." But from where I was standing, it seemed like the world was going to come to an end. My sense is that if she had had more experience putting a number to her feelings, she would have chosen a "10."

She walked up the stairs.

She didn't count.

She was a wreck.

And she remained a wreck for most of 10 minutes. Just lingering with her feelings. My job was to be there with her and help her to refocus her thoughts back to how she was feeling about not counting the stairs. I had seen that terror in her eyes before. It was brutal.

Dr. Lang gave us a form to fill out.

We did it once a day for a week:

Counting Stairs Exposure/Response Prevention Homework						
Day	Start	1 Min	2 Min	5 Min	10 Min	15 Min
Tue	7	7	6	4	3	
Wed	8	7	6	3		
Thu	4	3	2			
Fri	No reaction					
Sat	9	8	5	2		
Sun	5	3	2			
Mon	4	3	2			

Notice that it got better as time went on. And the terror didn't last as long.

This was amazing.

Within a few more days, she was fine. Whenever we went up or down some stairs, I'd ask her if she had counted them. "No" *Did you think about it?* "Yes." *Did it bother you?* "No."

We did the same thing with the crossing light. I'd drive her to within a hundred feet of the crosswalk and let her out of the car. She'd walk up to the light, press the button—just once—then wait to cross. (I couldn't believe she had a 100% success rate for getting the light to change on just one press—I always thought it took more than that.) After she crossed the street, I'd pick her up, we'd fill out the form, and then get back to whatever we were doing—usually fleeing from an urge to cut.

The next step was to apply this to cutting. Dr. Lang talked with her professors and designed an exposure protocol they were willing to try. They wanted me to be a part of it. They asked Patricia and me for permission to videotape it. We agreed.

The next meeting with Dr. Lang was unreal. When we arrived, one of her medical school professors—a prominent Worcester child psychologist and member of the group I'd identified as one you'd like your kid to see—but who was inaccessible to the masses—was sitting in Dr. Lang's office holding a video camera. He was there just in case something went wrong. And to videotape it. Dr. Lang would do the rest.

The plan was to do three exposures that day. They would do the first one by themselves—with me safely ensconced in the waiting room. If everyone survived, I would get to witness the second one. The third time, I'd get to do it while they watched.

I was summoned back to Dr. Lang's office about 20 minutes into the hour. All three of them—Patricia included—had pleased smirks on their faces.

Then they put on a show for me. They explained that Patricia's job was to think about her urge to cut and not distract herself or change the topic. The doctor's mission—and ultimately mine—was to help Patricia stay on task by talking about the urge to cut. Again, she had some "bossing back clues." Just two this time:

1)   She can take deep breaths;
2)   She can talk about her urge to cut.

Period.
I folded my hands. They started.

DISCLAIMER: You should know by now that I am not a doctor. Please go back and reread the medical disclaimer on the copyright page. Do not try this at home. There were four of us in the room as this was happening: me, Patricia, and two doctors. One of them was there specifically to rescue us if things went badly. I have left out much of the meaty parts.

Urge to Cut Exposure Dialogue		
Time	Dr. Lang	Patricia
0:00	I want you to focus about the thought that you want to cut. Do you have the urge now?	Yes.
0:07	OK. What are you thinking about?	I need to cut.
0:10	You need to cut? How strong is it?	7.
0:13	It's a 7. OK. So tell me what you are thinking about.	I need to use a razor and cut my legs.
0:19	What are you going to use?	A razor. Or pinch myself.
0:24	You want to pinch yourself and you want to use a razor.	I want to pinch myself.
0:29		

This goes on ... and on ... for pages ...

		2.
2:41	You want to pinch yourself.	I want to bite myself.
2:44	You want to bite yourself. Are you thinking about wanting to cut right now?	I want to cut myself.
2:50	OK. Keep thinking about it.	[Nod.]
2:53	You want to cut yourself. Keep thinking about it. What is your temperature right now?	1.
2:57	I think we can probably stop.	

The urge to cut was gone.

Gone.

For the first time in years.

It took 2 minutes 57 seconds to make a feeling go away that had been haunting her for years.

Incredible.

The conversation with the doctors later was bizarre. They admitted that what they were saying made no logical sense. We talked about what I had just witnessed.

We talked about the difference between talking about the urge to cut and rationalizing about it. They assured me that they weren't trying to talk Patricia out of cutting. They were just trying to sustain the urge for as long as possible without thinking about something else.

They tried to convince me that Patricia wasn't doing anything to make those numbers lower. Her brain was doing it. The only thing she did voluntarily was concentrate really hard and tolerate feeling cruddy (which she was quite good at). While she was doing that, her brain chemistry was changing and rebalancing itself so it no longer focused on the feeling. They explained that this was happening at a brain level. Involuntarily. Breaking previous chemical and electrical associations between the thoughts and what her brain and behavior was. And actually, rational discussion would accidently strengthen the OCD symptoms. They wanted Patricia to just focus on the urge to cut and not on how she felt about it. And to keep focused on the intense, discomforting thought. Or the urge.

They acknowledged it was illogical. They likened it to torture.

That's what it looked like to me.

But it worked.

It worked for me when I tried it a few minutes later.

It worked for Tara after she'd seen the video and agreed to assist Patricia with it when she was at school.

And every time Patricia did an exposure, the relief she got from not having an urge to cut lingered for another hour. Or another day. Or another week.

It was incredible.

∞

But just because the urge to cut was becoming controllable didn't mean the dizziness was any better. Patricia continued to stumble around. She was grabbing onto the furniture to get from place to place around the house. She fell when she got up at night to use the toilet (because of all the water she was drinking). She passed out getting off the bus at school.

Because Dr. Goodman was on vacation, we went to see his covering psychiatrist. He took one look at Patricia's medication list and announced that her dizziness was because of too much Clozapine. Way too much Clozapine. So he reduced it.

When that didn't work, Dr. Fitzgerald sent us to see a neurologist in Worcester. He sent Patricia to Boston for some fancy balance tests—vestibular testing—to see if something was going on with her inner ear. There wasn't. But after the appointment, Patricia and I went downtown for lunch at Quincy Market, a popular tourist destination in Boston. As I held her hand to help her down the steps, she said, "Oh, look. A kiosk. Maybe we should take a picture and show it to [my old middle-school English teacher]. She's never heard of these."

Even through her stupor, she was able to hold onto that grudge for years.

Patricia was getting behind in school. She had stopped doing homework. And she wasn't awake enough to care. Normally, blips in schoolwork would be the fuel for her anxiety. Nothing.

Her teachers were worried. She hadn't learned anything new in the last month. And she couldn't repeat back anything she had learned in the last six. Finals were next week. They started talking about giving her an Incomplete in all her classes and finishing them up in the summer.

Patricia didn't care.

Dr. Goodman came back from vacation. We made an appointment for the next day. *Gee, it didn't take weeks to get in to see him.*

I'm the one who had been writing stuff down for the last three years. I knew the timing on the Luvox and Clozapine was all wrong. They weren't causing the dizziness. Not one of these doctors seemed to care that I knew it started with the Naltrexone. I was sure of it. *Sort of.*

This time, instead of beating around the bush or asking leading questions with the hope he would think about the Naltrexone as a possible cause for Patricia's dizziness, I decided to try something new: The direct approach. I handed Dr. Goodman a handwritten note as we began our appointment:

Father requests permission to stop Naltrexone.

1) It isn't working.
2) It's the only medicine added as dizziness symptoms started that hasn't been reduced.

Dr. Goodman stopped the Naltrexone.

The next day, Thursday, was the start of finals. Patricia's teachers refused to let her take the two scheduled for that day. Patricia was happy to stay home and sleep. The same thing happened on Friday. Except she didn't sleep through the whole day. She was up and around. Not bumping into things. Not falling down.

On Monday, about a hundred hours after stopping the Naltrexone, a newly awake Patricia aced that day's finals. She did the same thing Tuesday. And she made up the three missed ones within a couple of days.

She finished everything that semester.

Except *A Tale of Two Cities*.

(7772) (7772) (7772) (7242) (CG596) (CG596) (12 25)

+ (7772)

Finishing High School

If I were writing the new DSM-5, I would add a new illness called PLS, Patricia Larsted Syndrome. Or maybe Place Last Seen. Everyone growing up experiences it to some degree. It starts with anxiety, progressively adds depression, obsessive-compulsiveness, and ultimately, psychotic features. How much it affects each of us is related to one thing: loss of control and all its nuances—trauma (either real or imagined), neglect, bullying, difficult friendships, sickness—you know, childhood; and our ability to cope with it. Growing up cures it. But only if we make it that far.

∞

It took another year for Patricia to graduate from high school. We didn't realize it until it was over, but the agenda for that time was essentially built on the substance of the week-long report we prepared for Dr. Lang. We were so excited about the self-diagnosis of OCD, which led to the successful CBT exposures, we neglected to remember all the other things happening during that week. And because it wasn't so different from the hundred before it, I sometimes wonder if we could have short-circuited Patricia's illness and started work on restoring her life a little sooner if we had just been more aware of what was going on with her. Maybe The Quest wasn't all about her, but what others saw in her.

There was an IEP meeting bright and early Tuesday morning of that week. Patricia slept through most of it because we had spent until three a.m. at EMH figuring out it's OK to have thoughts of suicide as long as you don't have an actual plan. In the morning, I sat next to her at the table so whenever she slumped over too far or needed to say something, I could just nudge her with my shoulder. She managed to participate and give the illusion of keeping up.

That meeting was the beginning of a year-long project to get Patricia some real testing to try to understand how her brain worked. Although we met with the school and the district at least once each year to review and make minor adjustments to Patricia's IEP, a comprehensive review is only scheduled every third year. The problem was that the first IEP meeting was held during the fall of her sophomore year, which meant the next one wasn't scheduled until six months after she was supposed to graduate. I asked if we could move that meeting to the upcoming spring so Patricia would leave high school with a shiny new IEP—just in case one might be useful wherever she ended up. The school district agreed. And, amazingly, they also agreed to do some more psychoeducational testing so we all might better understand her learning style and abilities. My goal was to make her last year of high school as productive as possible. She had missed so much. And she continued to miss out on more every day.

At every opportunity, I had been asking Patricia's doctors and schools why it was that when she took high-stakes exams, she tested better at math than at English. No one had ever been able to explain it. Her teachers always labeled her as a prolific reader and a gifted writer, yet her testing scores didn't reflect it. She had done the same thing on her SATs, but with the added complication of both scores being significantly lower than anyone expected.

Patricia was in a better place emotionally as she went through this new testing. We ended up with another big report, one we thought did a pretty good job of describing Patricia: Very bright. Very anxious. There were all kinds of complicated details describing all the tests and sub-tests they had put her through. It said she had incredible cognitive abilities, both verbal and non-verbal, but especially verbally. Working memory—not so good. In fact, way below average.

The report acknowledged my question about high-stakes testing, but never answered it. It only addressed the disparity between the state MCAS tests and the SATs. It said Patricia requires familiarity in order to excel. We always knew Patricia would stand back and look at what the other kids were doing before she was willing to join in. Apparently, Patricia did better on the MCAS tests than on her SATs because she had been taking them every year since third grade. Maybe her SAT scores would improve each time she took them over again.

If she took them again.

Patricia announced she was happy with her SAT scores and would not be taking them again.

When it was time again for Patricia's annual physical, I lamented to Dr. Fitzgerald about my unanswered math/English question. She asked if we ever had any real neuropsychological testing done. *Not really. We had psychoeducational testing.* Not the same thing. Dr. Fitzgerald said to get it done. Incredibly, the insurance company agreed to pay for it.

We spoke with one of the "good" testers in town who agreed to build on the school testing by adding some new tests, including some "projective" ones. This meant that for the first time, they would add inkblot and other personality tests to the normal battery of "objective tests," which are the normal part of IQ testing. Patricia spent a couple of sessions with the doctor.

A couple of weeks later, there was a Report. And for the first time, it got our kid right. It described exactly what we had been living with for the last 17 years. All the little nuances of how she saw the world—and tried—and sometimes failed—to fit into it.

It was devastating.
But it was honest.

And once again, just like with the psychiatrist from Patriot Medical, the best part of The Report wasn't what was written down, but the conversation with the doctor after she handed it to me. She described her reinterpretation of the results of the psychoeducational testing done by the school earlier in the year. She focused on the huge differential in the IQ subtest scores, particularly between the verbal comprehension, perceptional reasoning, working memory and visual memory. For a typical child, these differences would indicate a Non-Verbal Learning Disability. But because Patricia's scores were overall so strong, she couldn't put that in her report—because if she did, her colleagues would drum her out of the neuropsychological testing business.

She described an individual whose working memory couldn't keep up with the rest of her brain. One who had trouble seeing the big picture, but who did a brilliant job of doing something—just not necessarily what the instructions were trying to get her to do.

This was Patricia.

And it began to answer my math/English question, too. Because with high school math, particularly early high school math, you don't spend a lot of time wallowing in the big picture. All you need to do is answer the question. But with English, particularly English composition, you need to think about the point you want to get across; develop a narrative with a beginning, middle, and end; and then put it all down on paper. So that someone else understands your understanding. Of the big picture.

This reminded me of the tomato planter fiasco. It started with me buying one of those "As Seen on TV" hanging bags filled with dirt with a tomato plant coming out the bottom. I wanted Patricia to assemble it so she could experience the thrill of accomplishing something. *Bad idea.* Because trying to safely add soil to a bag with a delicate plant coming out the bottom—a plant being crushed by the weight of the new soil being loaded at the top—was more than she could plan and execute. She could read the directions. But she didn't understand that if she smashed the fragile plant, the whole effort would be wasted. The point of the exercise was to end up with a living tomato plant, not just a bag of dirt.

The Report also included a suggestion to include some social skills training in Patricia's treatment plan. She recommended a book by Jed Baker entitled *The Social Skills Picture Book for High School and Beyond*. There were pictures of kids in a school setting with examples of the right way—and wrong way—to interrupt in class and deal with friendships. It reminded me of the kind of book you might see in preschool; except the pictures were of high schoolers instead of toddlers.

The day it arrived, I had it with me in the car when I picked up Patricia at a bus stop near her school. When she got into the car, she started ranting about the kid who had been sitting next to her on the bench—smoking—even though there was a NO SMOKING sign posted right there. The smoke didn't bother her; it was his blatant disregard for the rules that was making her nuts. I put the car in park, opened the book up to page 98, and made her read the section called "Don't Be the Rule Police" as we sat there and watched him enjoy the rest of his cigarette.

When she finished, she thanked me for pointing out that it really wasn't her fault that he was ignoring the sign. (I'm not sure she believed what she was saying.) The book is filled with examples of how to get along in society—things she never learned as she was growing up.

∞

During the IEP meeting, we talked about Patricia's graduation requirements. She was doing fine—Abenaki High had given her credit for everything she tried to do before leaving for The Steuben School, and she was picking up a whole semester of extra credits every summer. Gym and foreign language were the two problems. She solved gym by taking it twice a week during the fall of her senior year.

Foreign language was the bigger problem. The school district required two years. Technically, Patricia had credit for one and a half, even though there wasn't a lot of learning going on during the fall of her sophomore year. The Steuben School did not offer any foreign languages. Because of this, the district was willing to waive the requirement. They'd just let it slide. The problem is that most colleges require those two years. People at the table began to wonder if maybe the disability office at whatever college Patricia decided to go to might be willing to waive the requirement. Why not ask?

But Patricia wasn't prepared to play along with any of this. If her classmates back at Abenaki could complete two years of a foreign language, then so could she. She was unwilling to accept a waiver. Therefore, she needed another half year. Of Latin II.

The school suggested an online course. We knew how badly that went with the photography class Patricia and I took together. I was skeptical. They suggested a correspondence course from some place in Texas. *At least it's not online.* Patricia agreed. She took one semester of Latin II by mail. She tried to read the book. (It was in a foreign language.) She did the worksheets. (You know how much she likes those.) She mailed them off to a teacher halfway across the country. (Who took forever to correct and return them.)

Patricia's pretty good at math—so she calculated how long it would take her to finish the class if she waited for feedback from her teacher in Texas before starting on the next lesson—five years. So she signed my mother up to tutor her. After all, Latin hadn't changed in thousands of years—why would it have since grandma took it nearly half a century ago. They plodded through all the lessons, stuffed them in a big envelope, and mailed them off.

She passed. *Whew.*

∞

Worcester, Massachusetts is famous for just a few things: Triple-deckers. Robert Goddard, the father of modern rocketry. And the guy who invented the smiley face.

On December 3, 1999, Worcester became famous for a horrific building fire that killed six firefighters. It took days to put it out and recover their bodies. Our community was devastated.

When it came time for a memorial service, everyone came. Even the president. I took a couple of hours off work and walked downtown to watch the funeral procession. What struck me most were the 30,000 firefighters from around the world who came to pay their respects. Some were dressed in their best uniforms—polished buttons and crisp pleats. But most just showed up in the only thing they had—their turnout gear. The sight was incredible.

When it was over, as I walked back to work, I passed by the city's main fire station. Hanging on a chain-link fence were several hand-drawn posters. Messages from local school children to the lost firefighters. I slowed to read them.

I was struck by one:

"May your house be safe from tigers."

I burst into tears.

A few days later, I made my way down to the fire site. A makeshift memorial had sprung up nearby. A fire truck, parked by the side of the road, was festooned with mementos left by people coming to pay their respects. Flowers. More of those notes. Flags. T-shirts.

I collect things. I've been doing it for years. I call it "Real Word Stuff™." It started with sand from some of the beaches I've visited. It has grown into trying to collect some little something from the places I've been that will remind me of that special day. Some of the things are straightforward: Confetti from the millennium in Times Square. Water from The Great Salt Lake. A dining room table. Others are more esoteric: Light from a Leonid Meteor Shower. Fog from the Sargasso Sea. I keep some of the stranger stuff in little glass bottles I have for just this purpose.

As I walked up to the fire truck, I kept wondering how I could collect something that would remind me of this solemn place and time. I certainly wasn't going to take something someone else had left—that's not how I do it. Maybe I'd find some soot. Or maybe just a smell would be enough. As I came around the truck, in the back, amid all the flowers and the other stuff, was a baseball hat. With four letters embroidered on the front. FEMA.

It took my breath away. I burst into tears again.

I went back to my car, opened the glove compartment, took out two of my little bottles, and walked back to the fire truck. One by one, I opened each, filled it with my breath, and sealed it up again. I left one on the truck's bumper. The other went into my pocket.

Some things are bigger than one person, or one family, or one community can handle. For Worcester, it was that fire. We needed the whole country to support us. And they came.

Mental illness, like fires, strikes at unexpected times and in unexpected places. The victims and those trying to support them aren't always in the best position to be able to handle it themselves. And even if they don't always know the right thing to do, sometimes, we need our government to throw its hat into the ring, too. To help us make our houses safe from tigers.

∞

Maybe Latin wasn't changing. But I was. And it wasn't by choice. During one of my parent support group speaker meetings, I learned about the four stages of dealing with a traumatic life event: "denial," "anger," "acceptance," and finally, "advocacy." I listened with casual dismissiveness knowing that advocacy wasn't a part of me or something I would ever consider doing. I wasn't willing to talk about what was going on with Patricia with anyone, let alone advocate for her—or anyone else for that matter—in a public setting. I don't talk to people. *Or do I?*

But something happened. And it made me mad. I learned that CAP, the Collaborative Assessment Program, the program that had saved Patricia's life by getting her access to the people at the Department of Mental Health, had been discontinued. It was being replaced with something else. And the problem was that this new program was only accessible to children who were covered by Mass Health, the new public health-insurance program being touted as Massachusetts's first experiment with universal healthcare. It's only available to low income families or to those "already in the system" for one reason or another. New families like mine with private insurance experiencing what Patricia went through would no longer be eligible for the emergency wraparound services that helped us to build the framework which enabled Patricia to survive. *This is stupid.*

And it's stupid on a bunch of levels.

Imagine coming home to find your house on fire and you lived in a society that had moved on from that ancient 911 system. Instead of just picking up the phone and calling 911, how you react is now dependent on the kind of insurance you have. If you have no insurance? Or Mass Health? 911 still works. They show up and put it out. But if you have private insurance, you need to find your policy, look up the section on house fires—only to find out that you need to know whether it is an electric fire, a stovetop grease fire, or a problem with the furnace, hypothetically—hard to tell through all the smoke—and then go online to look up all the different providers who are authorized to put out that kind of fire. After a quick pre-approval process, maybe in a couple of weeks, after a few unreturned phone calls, you finally learn your insurance company has agreed to authorize payment. All you have to do is get on the waiting list at one of those providers.

Your house has long since burned down. Your family is dead. It's too late.

So every time I heard that some commissioner or legislator was holding a meeting to hear about how things were going in their community, I showed up and talked about Patricia and how CAP saved her life. I told them how ridiculous it seems that if I were to do all this over today, the smartest thing for me to do would be to lose my job—so I would be eligible for Mass Health—just in case my child ever came down with a disease I couldn't pronounce. Then I looked them in the eye and told them it was going to be their fault when the next kid died because of their stupid program.

So far, they still haven't fixed it.

∞

Patricia managed to stay involved with Destination Imagination for yet another year. She was an assistant manager for two teams at her old elementary school. Her school bus got her back in town just in time to make it to their weekly after-school meetings. She felt needed. She was needed. After all, she had nine years of DI experience; her adult co-managers had never been on a team.

Both teams made it to the state finals.

Each year, Massachusetts Destination Imagination hands out several college scholarships. They encourage graduating seniors to apply. The running joke is that in order to win one, you need to write an essay that will make the state director cry as she reads portions of it aloud during closing ceremonies at the state tournament. Patricia decided to write about her troubled adolescence and to credit DI with keeping her alive through those difficult years. She won a scholarship. The big one. The director cried.

Massachusetts DI also gives out a special tassel to all the high school seniors to wear on their mortarboards at graduation. This, more than anything else, is her most cherished prize from her DI years.

∞

In addition to the visit to EMH one night during the week of the Dr. Lang report, a few months later there was another hospitalization. But this time it was only for a couple of days. As always, it still took hours to get admitted, but it was a calm and controlled operation. We were dealing with people at both EMH and Six West who were familiar with Patricia and her struggles. Ultimately, her medicines needed to be bumped back up to the therapeutic level where they had been before everyone started slashing them during The Time of Dizziness.

Patricia was getting older. I was getting sick of doling out her medications. She was on so many that it took a big chunk of my Sunday afternoon to organize a week's worth of her pills. We used a weekly pill organizer tray with seven daily snap-out pill cases, each with four covered compartments. The tray lived in the locked medicine safe. One came out each day.

Patricia did a remarkably good job of remembering to take them at the right time. But she wasn't always consistent about taking the right ones. Twice in one week, the school called to say Patricia thought she had taken her nighttime pills by mistake that morning. She had fallen asleep more than normal on the bus. I checked, and sure enough, she was right. In her morning stupor—which seemed to be getting worse and lasting longer every day—Patricia would pick up her pill case, open the compartment on the end, dump the pills into her mouth, and dry-swallow them. *Yuck.* But she had opened the wrong end. We moved the "Bed Time" pills down one hole and the problem went away.

Teaching Patricia to fill the pill cases herself was a disaster. It was like an engineer trying to explain rocket science to a toddler. I wanted her to count the pills as she took them out of the bottle, listen to the sound as each dropped into its compartment, and count again to confirm that everything was correct. She would take a handful and sprinkle them in. I asked her if she had gotten it right. She said, "Yes." I asked her to recount them. She did. I asked if she was sure they were right. She said, "Yes."

She was always wrong. *Wasn't needing to count things part of Patricia's OCD?*

It took months to get her to slow down enough to get a week right for the first time. It took even more months for her to get it consistently right. Maybe I'm just a bad teacher.

∞

It was time to think about graduation. Patricia had passed the MCAS tests, a requirement for getting a high school diploma in Massachusetts. She was making progress on her IEP goals, and like *Mental Health, The Musical,* The Steuben School only had so much to teach her. Convincing the school district to keep her in a therapeutic high school for another year past her normal graduation date was going to be a hard sell. (No one told me until after she graduated that teaching her to function in the real world is the job of the school district before they give her a diploma.) So I was prepared to let it happen. She was looking forward to graduating on schedule with the rest of her friends.

College was next. It was on that list for Dr. Goodman.

As I talked with Patricia about what kind of colleges she wanted to visit, it was clear she had done some thinking and had made some decisions for herself. The most important one was that she wanted to commute from home—at least for her first year. Luckily, we live within 10 miles of a dozen first-rate colleges. When the ones for engineers, doctors, and veterinarians got crossed off the list, she had a choice between the local community college and the state university.

Patricia visited both. She called each up, signed up for a tour, and went. I got to drive and tag along. This was new—not the tour—she had been on one of those with a couple of classmates from school—but the her-calling-up part.

After the tour of the community college, as we sat in the car getting ready to come home, I asked Patricia how our tour was different than the one she had taken with her school. She thought for a minute and said, "Today's tour was led by a regular student; the other one was by a student from Disability." Although she had seen similar things, her previous tour also included peeks into the disability office and another room, a large, quiet room, filled with computers, which the guide said was reserved for disability students, like him, and was where he spent much of his free time.

We checked our campus map, found the disability office, walked over, and barged in. Patricia said hello, told them she had been on a tour today, that she was thinking about applying to their college, and she was interested in learning about their disability services. We left with another pile of brochures and the offer to make an appointment to come talk about what kind of accommodations she might need. The secretary whispered to me that Patricia had done a great job of advocating for herself.

We did the same thing at the state university. She came home with nearly as many brochures.

The only one missing from the second batch was this form; the one I thought was the best of all:

Who Am I in 5 Steps

Student Name:

What is your Disability?

1. How does it impact your learning?

2. What are some of your academic strengths?	**What are some of your academic weaknesses?**

3. What Accommodations have you used in the past?

☐ Extended time to take tests
☐ Taking tests in location separate from the class
☐ Scribe to help with written assignments or tests
☐ Calculator for math or science
☐ Note-taking assistance / Handouts or copies of teacher notes
☐ Preferential seating in the classroom
☐ Access to specialized tutors or teachers
☐ Tests rewritten or reformatted
☐ Assistive Technology – specify:
☐ Books and other materials in a different format

      Circle one: Audio   Enlarged   On a computer

☐ Interpreter of American Sign Language
☐ C-Print Captioning
☐ Closed Captioning
☐ Computer for exams
☐ Other – specify:

4. What works?
Which of these accommodations worked best for you? Why?

Which of these accommodations do you use the most?

Is there anything you did not use but think might be helpful in college?

This is great. Unlike the SSRI Suicide Checklist, this thing actually tries to understand what works and how to set yourself up for success. The problem is that it only works if the prospective student knows how to answer the questions. And I questioned if Patricia actually had the answers. It wasn't going to work if I filled it out for her. I also decided that this form was the foundation of whatever plan Patricia must have in order to have any chance of succeeding in college. We talked about it. For six weeks. Every time I brought it up, I was careful not to have the form in front of me. I wanted to know what Patricia had been thinking about. Unfortunately, the answer was "nothing."

I signed up Tara to help. She, well, actually, he—because we were on the third version of Tara by now because the other ones had moved along to greener pastures after their therapeutic-high-school-counselor stints and so Tara was now a he—agreed to help Patricia fill it out.

I was pleased it came out differently than if I had done it. I expected the testing-in-a-separate-location checkmark. I was intrigued by the preferential-seating checkmark. It turns out Patricia likes to sit in the front corner of the classroom. If she never looks around, she can pretend she is the only one in class. *For a kid who doesn't like to be the only one in the class?* Patricia added two other possible accommodations: Access to a clinician when she was anxious or distracted by the voices. And listening to music on her headphones during tests. It drowns out the voices.

Most insightful were Patricia's answers to the other questions on the form. She was able to acknowledge many academic strengths: a fast, prolific reader; an accomplished writer and poet; computer savvy—able to Excel®; and, with support, able to excel. She also admitted to some weaknesses: trouble with standardized testing; a lousy math foundation from fast-tracking in middle school; and excess personal drive, causing her to pace herself faster than she can learn, even when her illness prevents her from concentrating. *Wow.*

The result of all of this, Patricia concluded, was a history of shutting down and freaking out during times of anxiety brought on by stress or the voices. Time made it better. So did access to a clinician and the milieu of a therapeutic school, something she knew neither prospective college could offer.

Patricia applied to both places, the community college and the state university. After careful thought, she decided to check the box on the application asking to be considered for the "special admissions opportunity as an applicant with a documented learning disability." She included a copy of her most recent psychoeducational testing, just like the instructions said.

Getting into a community college in Massachusetts is easy. Anyone with a high school diploma gets in. Patricia was on track for that, so they were happy to talk with her. She signed up for a meeting with the disability office, made a copy of her Who Am I in 5 Steps form, and went to see them. When it was over, Patricia showed me her shiny new Accommodation Letter—they had granted several on the spot, including everything she wanted, except for the listening-to-music-while-taking-tests one. They said they had no way to control what she was listening to.

Getting into the state university took six weeks. Patricia was very pleased. She knew a number of people who had been rejected. Deciding where to go was another project. Patricia was all set with the community college. All she needed to do was to stop by the campus, take some placement tests, and sign up for classes. Making a decision about the state university wasn't as easy. The question Patricia needed to answer was whether or not the university could provide her the supports she needed in order to succeed. She already had a positive answer from the community college. So she called them up and tried to make an appointment with the disability office.

They refused.

They said that because she was not an enrolled student, they would not talk with her.

This is ridiculous.

I fumed about this for a few days.

But if they wouldn't talk to her because she wasn't enrolled, why not just pretend to enroll? It cost me $150. I wrote the check. She could always change her mind. They agreed to speak with her. They promised to let her know by sometime in May—June at the latest—what day she could come in and meet with someone in the disability office. But it wouldn't be until the summer.

This is ridiculous.

All Patricia wanted to know was that that they had looked at the psychoeducational testing she had included with her application, they were comfortable that the university was equipped to provide a supportive environment, and she would have a good chance of succeeding.

Please understand that this is all written with a straight face. This is not meant to be funny. I believed that there was an answer to this question. Actually, there was.

It took Patricia a couple of months to figure out that she got into college because of her SAT scores, school grades, essay, and all the other stuff that is part of a regular college application. No one looked at her psychoeducational testing. Nobody cared that Patricia checked off the disability box on the application.

Unfortunately, this also meant that no one had given any thought to whether or not Patricia might be able to handle it.

The decision was left up to her.

Ultimately, she chose the university over the community college because she read in one of their brochures that the disability office would help her sign up for the right classes. I decided not to tell her that the community college brochure, which she never read, said the same thing.

The other thing Patricia learned when it was almost too late is that there is a difference between the disability office and the counseling office. Patricia had spent the last two and a half years at a therapeutic school with unlimited access to a clinician. And backup clinicians. That meant she had someone she could go talk to who would help put her back together when things weren't going very well. Over those years, Patricia accessed these resources many times each day.

Patricia and her parents were surprised to learn that this is the job of counseling, not disability. The job of disability is to grant reasonable accommodations for students with documented learning disabilities and to provide a letter for each teacher to read and handle in whatever way they chose. Counseling puts the kid back together, if possible, but only if someone happens to be available.

Unlike public schools, where each child is entitled to a free and appropriate education in the least restrictive environment—despite disability—there is no such promise after graduating high school. And unlike public school, there is no requirement for teachers to provide extra help or change expectations just because of a disability. Patricia was expected to learn everything her classmates would be learning—at the same pace—and without disrupting the class in any way that might deny her classmates the learning opportunity they were entitled to.

The real thing Patricia finally learned is that she was responsible for putting herself back together when things weren't going as well as she wished. It wasn't up to counseling. Or disability. It was up to her. They could help. But they wouldn't do it for her.

Nice to know.

Ultimately, Patricia hooked herself up with both the disability office and the counseling office before the first day of class. She used, and needed, both.

∞

The characters showed up again. They were playing Russian Roulette. It took a couple of weeks for the first one to die (and then hundreds of times again, because the stories play over and over again). Of all the characters, one of them was most like Patricia. She had been wondering for a while whether this character represents her own self. And then she began to wonder what might happen if this "self" died by her own hand in one of these stories.

Dr. Goodman brought up the possibility of ECT again. He wasn't exactly suggesting it, but he wanted it on the table so if or when it became appropriate, we wouldn't be surprised.

A couple of months later, he asked me to research TMS, Transcranial Magnetic Stimulation. It's a kind of therapy that uses a powerful magnet, like a small MRI, to stimulate just one part of the brain. He was having good results with lifting the depression of some of his more difficult patients.

And then another kind of voice started showing up. Unlike the "characters," these voices didn't have a persistent or recognizable personality. They just started talking. Mostly, all they did was a lousy job of predicting the future.

"The school is going to catch on fire. You won't be able to get out."

"Someone will come in with a gun."

I learned about them one day when Patricia and I were fleeing. We were driving down the Massachusetts Turnpike. As we approached a bridge, Patricia said, "A truck on the overpass is going to land on us." *What?* "A truck on the overpass is going to crash and land on us. That's what they are saying?" *Who?* "The voices." *What voices?* "The ones that are telling me that."

We managed to have a conversation about this.

I talked about the decisions I make every day when I drive. As I approach an overpass, I assess the situation and make sure it is safe for me to go under it. I look at the roadway to make sure it is clear and that nothing overhead might fall. I do it hundreds—probably thousands—of times, every time I drive. My point was that thinking about this stuff is normal. Maybe Patricia didn't understand that catastrophizing everything is a necessary part of being safe. I mentioned this to Patricia.

She said the difference between me and her was that I could move on. She would still be thinking about it a minute later. An hour later. Or maybe even a day later.

Maybe having an OCD-based anxiety disorder is just being more thorough.

We had known about Patricia's voices for years. When the doctors found out they were a problem, they wanted them gone. No one was ever interested in why they were around or what they were saying. Because we were trying to understand the root of what was going on with Patricia when we needed to do an exposure, we began to understand that what they were talking about was related to what was going on with Patricia.

The idea of including the voices in the conversation never came up. Except. Except that last day with Deb, just before she disappeared forever, they gave each voice a name and told them to go away. It worked. Why no one thought to try that again is beyond me.

Even after Patricia tried it again. And it worked.

One morning when the bus was late picking Patricia up for school, the characters showed up to let her know that the bus had broken down. She told them, "No, it hasn't. Go away." They went away. And stayed away. For a long time. That was the second time.

Including the voices in recovery is a game-changer.

∞

Patricia's CBT exposures became a big part of her life. She did them at home with me and at school with the new Taras. These provided significant and long-lasting relief from her urge to cut. Unfortunately, Patricia was more likely to spend hours being miserable, using her DBT coping skills, rather than recognizing that doing an exposure would actually make her feel better. It was always someone else's idea to do the exposure. It always worked. And the relief was always sustained.

We knew that stress and anxiety are what set Patricia off. We became good at figuring out how to avoid stressful situations, but the easiest was to stay home and doing nothing. And that caused its own problems. She'd get lonely; the characters would show up to keep her company; and then their stories would turn dark.

Accomplishing things was a different way to pass the time, and Patricia thrived on actually getting something done. She started using a "White Board." Every time she finished something, she'd write it down. It made her feel accomplished. Needed. Important.

We changed this around and began writing an agenda for the day—or the weekend—and then checking things off as she, or we, did them. Whenever I found her sitting at her desk waiting for someone to come online to chat, I'd redirect her to the white board for something else to keep her busy.

It worked.

But I never figured out how to help her remember that it was always sitting there on the dining room table. Waiting to be looked at. As she sat at her desk. Bored and lonely. With an urge to cut.

Because of my lack of social skills, I tend to talk in sound bites. Whenever it appears that someone has done something worthy, I say, "You're the greatest!" It makes me feel like I'm participating in life. Because I'm not very creative, I tend to repeat the same phrase over and over.

My most recent one was "What would Dorothy do?" I used this with Patricia every time she came to me for help because she was consumed with the urge to cut. I'd just say, "What would Dorothy do?" Dorothy, in the story of the *Wizard of Oz*, always had the power to get home again. She just never knew it. Patricia, like Dorothy, now had the power to make the urge to cut go away. But like the white board sitting on the table, it never occurred to her. She'd start up her DBT distraction skills and spend hours being miserable, rather than remember she could do an exposure and make the feelings go away.

So the answer to my question really was, "Nothing." Because Dorothy didn't do anything until the Wizard reminded her she had the power all along. Patricia's success rate to self-identify the need to do an exposure was 0%. She never figured it out on her own.

I decided to see if I could be the wizard. I fired up my Internet connection and ordered a few custom silicone wristbands—like those cancer-awareness ones everyone wears—except with the word "EXPOSURE" on them. Patricia put one on her wrist next to all her other bangles. I knew that when Patricia got nervous, she fidgeted. And when she fidgeted, she started playing with the stuff on her wrists.

Her ability to self-identify the need to do an exposure went to 100%. First day. *Incredible.*

It turns out that when Patricia was younger, I communicated in sound bites, too. I made t-shirts for Patricia with a word or phrase printed upside down on the front. She was supposed to look down and read it. There were two I remember.

One said "Enunciate." Apparently she had been mumbling for longer than I had remembered.

The other was "Consider Your Customer." It seems she had been having trouble seeing the big picture, as well.

∞

The exposures became more intense. Scarier. One day, the voices showed up and told Patricia that she was going to kill herself. (They didn't tell her *to* kill herself; they were just making a prediction.) They told her how—she would cut deep on her wrists. We decided to do an exposure on "The urge to cut in order to kill myself." Patricia focused on the feelings. She was at a "9" for almost four minutes—a near record.

We continued the exposure. At seven minutes, the urge to cut was gone, but Patricia was still scared she might cut anyway. This had never happened before. Exposures had always fixed her. I was panicking. If we got in the car and went to EMH, we could never explain this to the guy in the striped pastel shirt. It would take them a week to get Patricia out of the dark place she was in.

So we changed what we were focusing on. We went from "The urge to cut," to "I want to kill myself." I directed Patricia back to experiencing the feelings associated with that. Within a minute, that urge went away, too.

But Patricia was still scared.

A few minutes later, Patricia told me the voices had just shown up and were telling her *to* kill herself. She said, "This is the first time they ever told me to do something." *Who is stronger? You or them?* "I don't know. They can take me over." "I wish I was still weak because then I could kill myself and make them go away. But I can't. Because I promised to be strong." (This was a command hallucination—the first one ever?)

We switched the exposure from "I want to kill myself," to "Listen to what the voices are saying and rate how loud they are." I redirected Patricia back to listening to them.

Two minutes later, the voices were gone.

But Patricia was still scared.

So we changed the focus to "How scared am I?" I redirected Patricia back to those feelings.

Twenty-seven minutes after the exposure started, Patricia was fixed. And not just sort of fixed. *Fixed.* She took a shower, sat down in front of the TV, watched her evening shows, and went off to bed. The next day, she was fine. And the day after that.

The relief lasted for several days before we needed to do another exposure.

We did all this with our new exposure sheet. We had long since abandoned the one we used that first day with the stairs. The 1, 2, 5 and 10 minute time periods weren't right for Patricia; it was usually shorter than that, and she would sometimes go up and down within a single minute. Here is our sheet from that day. The real one was messier:

Tue			Exposure Log				
7:37	:00	:15	:30	:45	:60	Notes	
0:	9					Focus: "Urge to Cut in Order	
1:	9					to Kill Myself"	
2:	9					"Why do I feel sad in the first	
3:	9		8	7		place?"	
4:	7		6	5			
5:	5	4				"Confused."	
6:	4	3	2	1		"No urge to cut because I'm	
7:	1					at a 4. But I think I might cut	
8:	1					anyway."	
9:	1			5			
10:	1/5	4	3	2	1	Focus: "I want to Kill Myself"	
11:	1/1						
12:	1/1						
13:	1/1				8	"Voices present: Kill yourself."	
14:	1/1/8	7	6	5		Focus: "Loudness of Voices"	
15:	1/1/5	4	3	2	1	"This is the first time they ever	
16:	1/1/1					told me to do something."	
17:	1/1/1					Who is stronger? "Wish I was	
18:	1/1/1					weak so I could kill myself and	
19:	1/1/1					make them go away."	
20:	1/1/1					"Still scared. I have nothing	
21:	1/1/1		8	9		left to focus on."	
22:	1/1/1/9					Focus: "How Scared am I?"	
23:	1/1/1/9			8			
24:	1/1/1/8	7	6	5	4 3		
25:	1/1/1/3	2	1				
26:	1/1/1/1						
27:	1/1/1/1						

Today's Events:	Voices in class: "Someone will come with a gun." Better. Then back: "Car will hit you." PRN. Gone.
Today:	Worse 1 2 (3) 4 5 6 7 8 9 10 Better

∞

Nietzsche (some German philosopher-guy) once said, "That which does not kill us makes us stronger."

Like a lightning rod, Patricia had a knack for attracting trouble. But in the process, she had become the most resilient person I've ever met. Every time Patricia got knocked down and kicked in the face by life, she would get up, change her tactics, and get right back in there. More often than not, she'd get knocked down again. But it was always by something different.

Gradually, Patricia's perception of these events shifted from feeling like a loser to recognizing that she had overcome her darkness. And persevered.

I wish I had her strength.

∞

Patricia finished *A Tale of Two Cities*.

She chose to graduate with her class at The Steuben School. Because she was technically a student at Abenaki High, she could have attended that graduation, as well. But she opted to mark this milestone alongside the 14 kids with whom she conquered high school, not the 400 others.

The ceremony was held in a room at the Town Hall, just down the street from the school. All 15 graduates and their families were there. The school chorus sang. Some of the teachers and administrators said nice things.

But the best part was the speeches.

Every graduate was given the opportunity to say something. Most of them did.

I got to hear more than a dozen stories, each of them different, from a young adult who had more insight into him or herself than I have ever experienced—or thought possible—in anyone. They were all deeply grateful to the school, and sometimes to their parents, for helping them to find their own way through a very difficult childhood.

Patricia's speech was brilliant.

Eighteen

It's a few minutes past midnight. Patricia turned 18 yesterday. She's upstairs. Sleeping. I checked. Just now. And last night, too. For the first time in a long time. I hope she hasn't forgotten the promise she made to me two and a half years ago: The one to wait until yesterday to kill herself.

I hope she actually changed her mind.

The calendar says she's an adult now. She spent yesterday filling out Release of Information forms. She did a bunch at school. And another pile at Dr. Goodman's office. For the first time— correctly—there were forms giving the school and each doctor permission to talk with her parents, too.

Ultimately, what happens next is up to Patricia. She's in charge; just like she's always been. But from here on, it's her story. She still has a big team of professionals who are ready to help, a whole bunch of supporters, and three amateurs. Who are willing to lend a hand. For as long as she needs it.

Lessons Learned

I remember the day Patricia was born. She was just a few minutes old. I was sitting in the hospital room. And in one hand, I was holding this really tiny child. Someone I had helped create.

As I sat there with her, all I could think about was how difficult it was going to be to teach her—before she needed to know—about how to survive on thin ice.

This was a skill I first practiced when I was nine.

It was winter, early December, and the lakes had just started to freeze over. My friends and I weren't very heavy, so we tended to venture out farther than our parents would have let us—had they been around.

So there I was, 25 feet from shore, when there was a sound, "crack," as the ice underneath me started to give way.

I hadn't gone to engineering school, yet, but I had a sense about the way things worked in the world. And I was pretty sure the sound I just heard was going to be the beginning of me drowning in the icy water. And I was pretty sure I would take a friend or two with me if they made the wrong decision and decided to help.

I managed to get flat down onto the ice. Arms out. Legs out. My nose touching the thin sheet that protected me from the deadly water below.

I learned a lot about physics that day. As I put different pressures on each body part, the sounds the ice made changed. As I slid toward shore, I noticed the ice was getting thinner—maybe something to do with sunlight warming the shallow lake-bottom.

And when the ice finally broke, as we all know it was destined to do, I was able to crawl through the cold water the rest of the way to shore.

Sitting with Patricia that day in the hospital, I already knew there were things she was going to need to learn on her own. But I also knew she would be in a better position to survive these things if she had great exposure to the ways of the world.

Over the years, I did my best to give her those opportunities.

And she used them to amaze me.

∞

Patricia's journey isn't over. But this is a good place for us to stop and take a look back at what's happened. The bad. And the good.

About a year into this, Judy, my parent support group facilitator, asked me to come speak to a bunch of child psychiatry fellows from the local teaching hospital. The subject was supposed to be "a parent's perspective of clinician interactions in the adolescent mental health system." I wondered why she thought of me. And then I remembered all the stories she'd heard me tell about those bumpy clinician interactions.

My first reaction was, "ABSOLUTELY NOT!" I had spent my entire life avoiding speaking in public—or to anyone for that matter. I was quite good at it. And except for the confidentiality of the parent support group setting, I wasn't ready to tell anyone about what had been going on with my kid. But so much had happened. I had learned so much. And I was at a point where I wouldn't wish my experiences over that year on any other parent. So I agreed to do it. With conditions.

Rather than the "Conversation" they wanted, they agreed to let me read from notes. And they agreed to give me the 20 minutes I figured it would take to tell my story. It took 30. By the end, except for a couple of doctors, the whole room was in tears. One of the fellows tried to apologize to me for how I'd been treated by the medical community. But I started my story then—as I'll say again now—with the assertion that all the professionals we had dealt with, except for perhaps one, had truly tried to help Patricia. They certainly weren't all successful, but it wasn't because they hadn't tried. This remained true over the years. And I continue to appreciate everyone's efforts.

Because they would have my attention, I decided to add two more elements to my diatribe. One was my sister's idea. She recommended I finish up with a short list of take-aways for the fellows: Little pieces of advice that might help them as they begin their medical careers. I'll expand on that here, with some lessons for parents, professionals, educators, politicians, and survivors. Ultimately, I think I learned something for each of them.

My piece was to honor five of the heroes I'd met over the previous year. My life had changed so much during that time. And it really hadn't done so because of what I was doing, but because of little acts perpetrated by people around me. I recognized them during my Conversation with the fellows.

After the meeting, I decided to reach out to some of them and thank them personally for the difference they had made. Doing so forced me to put their part into the context of Patricia's story by sharing some of the details of what had been going on with her. And with me. I wrote each a letter, and presented them with a copy of my written remarks along with a little memento: a sandstone "Hero" medal I had made for the occasion. If you ever come across one out there in the world, know that you are in the presence of someone who made a huge difference in someone's life.

I gave one to a father who shared the story of his lost child.

I gave one to a doctor who asked me if I was all right when we were talking about something else.

I gave one to another doctor who worked to solve the real problem and not what the patient came in for.

There are two more I've been saving. They will find their homes at the appropriate time.

The first one had been intended for the receptionist at the psychiatrist's office. She's the one person who said, "Yes," when we needed it the most during those difficult early months. I was never able to give it to her because she moved from reception to a different job in the back office. I never saw her again. But because I had already written a glowing letter to her boss thanking him and his staff for saving Patricia's life, and because I had singled her out as an important part of his team, I decided not to track her down.

Ultimately, I'm glad I made that decision. Because it took me a couple of years to figure out that the real credit goes to the doctor himself. He's the one who surrounded himself with a caring staff who treats patients in the same way he did. Knowing when to fit the sick kid in sometime later today saved Patricia's life several times. He's the real hero. The medal will go to him.

The last one is for Patricia. She's my hero. Then. Now. And always.

For Parents

1) Make the phone call. Call back.
2) Talk to the kid.
3) Keep a log. Of everything.
4) Get over it. And then get on with it.
5) Use the coping skills you have learned.
6) Your kid might be sick even if they choose to deny it.
7) Your kid might be sick even if you choose to deny it.
8) The voices are real. Search for their meaning.
9) Make your spouse a partner in your child's treatment.
10) Advocate for your child.
11) Ask questions at the doctor's office.
12) Say thank you. Mean it.
13) Don't give up.

∞

For Doctors and Therapists

1) Return phone calls.
2) Talk to the kid.
3) Provide hope.
4) Fix sleep.
5) Never stop wondering if you have the right diagnosis.
6) Your patients are different. Treat them all differently.
7) Make sure the kid is getting services they need and not just ones you know how to provide.
8) Be honest. Don't sugar-coat anything.
9) Be the care coordinator if there isn't one.
10) If the voices are disruptive, make them go away.
11) Use times of recovery to build strength for relapse.
12) DBT's distress tolerance doesn't really fix anything. It just keeps your patient alive until you find something else that will.
13) There are several kinds of CBT. Make sure you are using the right one.
14) Hire office staff that treats your patients the same way you treat them.
15) Speak up.

For Educators

1) Talk to the kid.
2) Figure out what accommodations the student needs.
3) If the school environment is not safe, find a more appropriate one.
4) Implement the accommodations.
5) Be sure the accommodations are only crutches. Begin at once searching for ways to make them unnecessary.
6) Try not to change the expectations.

∞

For Politicians

1) Children can't be lumped into categories until you have enough information to know where to lump them.
2) Don't discriminate against private insurance.
3) Parent partners are an inexpensive way to save lives.
4) Make sure there is a care coordinator.

∞

For Survivors

1) Talk.
2) Find someone to confide in who can make a difference.
3) Be open and honest.
4) Bring a list of successes—and complaints—to your doctor. You will get better care.
5) When the meds work, live.
6) When the meds work, invest time making yourself stronger for when they stop working again.
7) Figure out what your one passion is and do everything you can to hold onto it.
8) Make a Wellness Journal. Show it to someone. Fill it with coping skills to get you through the tough times, but more importantly, make sure it includes things that actually make you feel better. Those are the things you are most likely to forget.

Author's Notes

I saw Rent again tonight—the movie this time. I wanted to take a second look at Mark to see if he really is the loser I made him out to be in the Parent Support Group chapter. Maybe he's not. During the first few seconds of the movie, he tells us he's thrown out the script and instead of trying to direct everything, he is just going to experience real life—something far more interesting than he could come up with on his own. And so Mark gets to live, too.

This story is inspired by real events. I write them as I choose to remember them. I've done my best on the dialog. Much is verbatim. Some I needed to make up. The sequence of everything is approximate. Some facts may be scrambled up in the wrong story. I've merged some characters together to simplify an already much-too-complicated history. My feelings are real.

As much as possible, this is supposed to be a story about Patricia. And maybe about me, too. I have tried to keep her mom and sister out of it. To protect them. The fact that Patricia's troubles were playing out while my wife was recovering from a serious stroke and my other daughter was trying to be a kid in the midst of terrible chaos made our story more challenging than I am able to describe here. Giving everyone the time and attention they deserved was an impossible task. I wasn't always successful, but I choose to believe that I tried.

The real hero behind this book is Patricia. She's the one with the resilience, who triumphed by overcoming impossible circumstances.

Thanks to Patricia and some of her doctors who helped me think about what very personal medical details were appropriate to include here. And what to leave out.

Thanks to Ann. To Lois. To Jane. To Meri. To my mother. To Molly. To friends—none of you abandoned us, which I now know is unusual. And to my employer. For allowing me the flexibility to be where I was needed most.

Many readers and Stuart Horwitz from BookArchitecture.com deserve the credit for the good parts of this book. The rest is what I was unwilling to change. Without their help, I would still be lost and without direction. Thank you all.

∞

Every one of those readers wanted to know what happed to Deb. But this is one of the problems with real life. I don't know. I left that one, last, desperate message on her answering machine.

She never called me back.

Last month, I tried to find her again. I called that same number and left another message. She returned my call within an hour. She isn't dead. I've mailed her a copy of the book. As she reads it, I hope she sees, as all my other readers have, that she is one of the good ones. She promised to call to schedule a time to get together for ice cream.

∞

One last story.

As I wrote this book, I thought it was just about Patricia and what she was going through. It turned out that it is also about me. And how I have changed. By a lot.

As high school was finishing up and Patricia was feeling a little better, she agreed to participate in some medical studies related to her illness. They asked me if I would be willing to participate, too, as the "healthy" relative. I reluctantly agreed.

Since then, as part of this and other studies, I've had an MRI, an EEG, blood work, neuropsych testing, a complete mental-health screening, and all kinds of other tests; all things I vividly remember watching Patricia suffer through during those early years. In addition to the good feelings associated with "giving back," I gained a fresh appreciation for Patricia and what she put up with. Neuropsych testing is hard. And intimidating.

Recently, those same testers called me up and asked if I was willing to participate in an expansion of that original study. They are investigating Cortisol, a hormone released by the body in response to stress, to see if it plays a part in bipolar disorder or schizophrenia. I said yes.

I drove to Boston and spent an afternoon spitting into a tube and having my heart rate and blood pressure checked as they put me through a gauntlet of tasks specifically designed to induce stress. I won't tell you what they did, but trust me, they are really, really good at it.

When it was all over, they wouldn't let me leave until the red drained from my face and I calmed down. After more than an hour, and after the doctor had checked my blood pressure for what seemed like the hundredth time, he finally said I could go. He handed me his business card and told me to give him a call if I ever had any questions or concerns. I stuffed it in my pocket and forgot about it.

But the next day, I dragged it out, called him up, and left a message.

When he called me back, I said something he wasn't expecting to hear. I told him that having been the caregiver for Patricia for all those years had changed me. And it had given me the strength to complete his study.

The old me never would have agreed to participate in the thing in the first place. I'd still be lurking in the back of the room.

The old me never would have called him back and left a message.

And that day in Boston, when he told me what that first task was, the old me would have died. Just died. On the spot. Right then. Dead.

But the new me finished that task. And the rest of them. And had fun doing it.

Having a sick kid changed me. For the better.

Epilogue

THE LIGHT

A play in one act.
Adapted for television.

SCENE: Dark.

The camera zooms out to reveal a darkened tunnel. A stone arch — regally emblazoned with the college name — supports the entrance. Ivy-covered buildings just begin to enter the scene.

From the dark, a face. Gradually, more and more of the walker is illuminated, lit only by the light entering the tunnel.

A college student, messenger bag over her shoulder, walks toward the camera. More students emerge from the darkness in the background. Walking. Obviously walking across campus.

Our walker: Eyes down. Then glancing up. Recognition. A slight smile ... very slight. Eyes back down.

She opens the passenger door and gets into the car.

FATHER: "How was your first day?"

PATRICIA: "I didn't die."

Extended pause.

FATHER: "Of what?"

PATRICIA: "Nerves."

Fade to light.

20732209R00139

Made in the USA
Lexington, KY
17 February 2013